The Forever Young Diet & Lifestyle

The Forever Young Diet & Lifestyle

James O'Keefe, MD, and Joan O'Keefe, RD

Andrews McMeel
Publishing

Kansas City

07 08 09 10 RR4 10 9 8 7 6 5

Library of Congress Cataloging-in-publication Data

O'Keefe, James H.
    The forever young and diet lifestyle / James O'Keefe and Joan O'Keefe.
        p. cm.
    Includes index.
    ISBN-13: 978-0-7407-5488-3
    ISBN-10: 0-7407-5488-2
      1. Longevity—Nutritional aspects. 2. Nutrition. 3. Diet. I. O'Keefe, Joan. II. Title.

RA784.O355 2005
613.2—dc22

2005053012

Book design by Holly Camerlinck

www.andrewsmcmeel.com

Attention: Schools and Businesses

Andrews McMeel books are available at quantity discounts with bulk purchase for educational, business, or sales promotional use. For information, please write to: Special Sales Department, Andrews McMeel Publishing, LLC, 4520 Main Street, Kansas City, Missouri 64111.

To my father, Judge James Henry O'Keefe Sr., who always kept his family at the center of his life and lived each day to its fullest. His passion for learning and writing, his cheerful discipline for fitness, and his Irish heart are the foundation upon which my world was built.

—JAMES

To my father, Leonard Olsen, a free and gentle spirit who greeted everyone with a smile and a song. His optimism, charm, and love of people and nature made me and everyone in his life feel special.

—JOAN

ACKNOWLEDGMENTS

Our families instilled in us love and interest for nature, fitness, health, spirituality, and service to others. This project is an outgrowth of those seeds. Our mentors at the Mayo Clinic strengthened those interests and showed us how to make a positive difference in the worlds of cardiology and nutrition. Our patients have taught us much, and they continue to inspire us each day. Psychologist Michael Bergman, a friend and fellow cyclist, provided insightful critical review of the material. Chris Schillig was invaluable in the editorial process; this project would not have come to fruition without her expertise. We feel privileged to be a part of the Cardiovascular Consultants at Mid America Heart Institute in Kansas City, an organization committed to excellence in patient care, research, and education. We would also like to thank Connie Smith and Jose Aceituno for their expert assistance.

CONTENTS

Part I: The Forever Young Diet . . . 1

Part II: The Forever Young Lifestyle . . . 175

The Forever Young Diet

1

INTRODUCTION

"Whatever you dream you can do—begin it.
Boldness has genius and power and magic in it."

—JOHANN GOETHE

By nature we are designed to be energetic, lean, fit, inquisitive, optimistic beings brimming with vim and vigor while living in the ideal native environment. Unfortunately, we are orphans of a world that is gone forever, and our environment is vastly different from that for which we were genetically designed. Staying healthy and fit doesn't come naturally to us anymore because some of our ancient and outdated instincts betray us. As adults we are "hard-wired" to move only when we have to, to rest when we can, and to eat as much as possible whenever food is available. Those instincts served us well in an untamed world where we had to save our energy in order to secure food, water, and shelter and withstand frequent periods of scarcity. If you follow these obsolete instincts in the ultraconvenient world of overabundance that is twenty-first century America, you will be doomed to a suboptimal life that includes obesity and illness.

The program detailed in this book combines the best of both the ancient and modern worlds. We will reintroduce you to the natural human diet and lifestyle, which has the power to bring you a lean body with forceful muscles and strong bones, an aerobically fit heart, a good immune system, and an attentive, curious, and confident mind geared toward working and playing harmoniously with others and building enduring social bonds. The program will also teach you how to take advantage of the greatest and safest modern pharmacologic breakthroughs. Often one or more of these drugs are needed as "correction factors" because we live in a world so foreign to our genetic makeup. You are living at the dawn of a revolution in the sciences of human health and aging. Scientists are learning how to engineer life itself, and the potential implications are vast and unparalleled. Much is yet to be discovered, but the basic tenets of how to achieve optimum health and longevity are clearly emerging. These principles are outlined in this book. They have the power to bring people longer, healthier, and more vigorous lives than any generation in the existence of the human race.

Yet most Americans, while living longer than their ancestors, are not living more vigorously. In fact, many people spend a large proportion of their life struggling with suboptimal and sometimes miserably poor health. Perceptive people are finally awakening to the urgency and gravity of this problem. The battle to achieve fitness and longevity in a high-tech, high-stress, high-calorie, inactive world that is conspiring to make us fat, sedentary, and lethargic can be fought and won one individual at a time, beginning with you. It is a high-stakes fight that you cannot afford to lose. This program is your battle plan for victory.

This book details a no-gimmicks program based on cutting-edge science. It contains practical, down-to-earth advice on how to become lean and youthful. There are currently 30,000 diet books available, yet most people don't know what to believe, how to eat, or what is right for their family. This book is about what works, not just for diet because nutrition alone is not enough to keep you lean, fit, and healthy for the rest of your life. The program also focuses on how to exercise and why you should embrace optimism, volunteerism, spirituality, and even have dogs and cats in your life. Here is a surefire way to rejuvenate your life and have fun in the process.

Find the Path Less Traveled

Many Americans are at a crossroads in their lives. By following the crowd in our inactive, junk-food society, we often find ourselves putting on a few extra pounds each year, and then struggling with yet another diet—only to fail once again. This path leads to a life drained of energy and enthusiasm that progresses to chronic illnesses and disability. After a decade or two on this diet and lifestyle, a person usually doesn't feel good or perform optimally and may barely recognize the face in the mirror some mornings.

However, you can choose to take the path less traveled. If followed closely, this course can revolutionize your health. You can regain a more youthful figure and improve your zest for life. Your outlook can be brighter and happier, and you will feel the energy coursing through your system. You will think more clearly, and decision making will seem easier. Your complexion will return to the vibrant glow of youth, radiating a natural beauty that comes from the inside out. You can turn back the hands of time and dramatically improve your overall health. Yet all the knowledge and technology in the world cannot help you make that transformation unless you are motivated and willing to embrace change.

We live in an environment that is in some ways toxic to our genetic makeup. Synthetic high-calorie food is everywhere—heavily marketed and delicious—leaving many of us powerless to resist its lure. To make matters worse, over the past 2.4 million years we are the first generation that modern technology has rendered physical activity entirely optional. Accordingly, almost two out of every three American adults are now overweight or obese, and fat has become the norm. The real question is not why so many of us are overweight but how anyone manages to remain thin in these surroundings.

Still, there is reason to take heart. You are a unique and special being, and you were meant to play an important role as our world unfolds. You have your own talents and perspectives, and the life around you will thrive best if you are self-actualized and fully engaged. In many respects there has never been a better place and time to be alive than America at the dawn of the twenty-first century. Life is full of opportunity and adventure, but in order to realize your full potential, you must start taking care of yourself. Your mind and body, even with their imperfections, are potentially among the most awesome, capable, and resilient entities in the known universe—make the most of these gifts.

If you view your body as your ally instead of your enemy, the healing and rejuvenation will begin. Caring for your body will become the priority instead of a second thought. You will find that you take pleasure in eating natural, highly nutritious, low-calorie foods like vegetables and fruits. Daily exercise will become second nature. Nothing succeeds like success, and you will find it easier with each passing day to feel respect and pride for your body as it grows stronger, leaner, and more youthful once again. Just vow to take the first step. Commit to making changes, and you will begin to feel and look better in hours to days, and soon this program will become self-perpetuating.

How to Switch Off the Aging Process

Natural selection is a cold and harsh process that is still culling the herd even in modern-day humans. Today, however, it will not be lions or wolves nipping at your heels and dragging you down. The modern predators are heart disease, cancer, osteoporosis, and the other diseases of aging. Your best protection against them is a physically active, emotionally connected lifestyle. Chris Crowley and Henry Lodge, MD, write in the superb book *Younger Next Year*: "In our forties and fifties our bodies switch into a 'default to decay' mode, and the free ride of youth is over. In the absence of signals to grow, your body and brain decay, and you age. What we can do, with surprising ease, is override those default signals, swim against the tide, and change decay back into growth. The keys to overriding the decay code are daily exercise, emotional commitment, reasonable nutrition, and a real engagement with living." These same principles form the foundation of the Forever Young program.

Mother Nature, in order to secure the future of the species, does her best to see that the youth will have enough food, resources, and space to thrive. Thus, after the childbearing and rearing years have passed, nature codes for the gradual demise of individuals who are no longer contributing to the well-being of the group as a whole. Seems pretty harsh, but here's the key: This age-related autodestruct mode can be switched off by signals that indicate continued viability and relevance of the individual to his or her surrounding life community. And whether or not you are still relevant is a judgment made by nobody else but you, though it may be at a subconscious level.

Staying physically fit, socially connected, and enthusiastic changes the hormones that resonate throughout your system to prevent aging and decay. You don't have to be engaged in negotiating world peace or discovering a cure for AIDS to stave off these decay messages. But you do have to do something that makes you feel as though you are still contributing. Become isolated, depressed, and idle and you are at risk for falling prey to the modern predators of natural selection.

Life is either in the growth mode or the decay mode; there is no middle ground. When you decide to sit back and aimlessly coast, and lose interest in pushing on, things start to deteriorate pretty quickly. Perhaps this is why humankind has always been so obsessed with finding "the meaning of life"—with it we stay young and vigorous; without it, we are programmed to begin to atrophy and die.

Who We Are

An old adage says "To those who do not hear the music, the dancers appear mad." We are often accused of being a little eccentric in our eating habits and lifestyle. However, if you want to be your best, we hope you will join us on the path less traveled. We guarantee that you won't regret it.

We have been passionate about nutrition and fitness virtually our entire lives, and we feel fortunate to be doing what we love—working in professions that promote health and healing. We met twenty-two years ago in the halls of St. Mary's Hospital of the Mayo Clinic in Rochester, Minnesota. At the time, James was a cardiology fellow, and Joan was completing her training in nutrition. As fate would have it, we stumbled across each other at the bedside of a gentleman with a bad heart and a serious weight problem, who needed both of our services. We hit it off immediately and have been best friends ever since. Our focus on health and diet was sharpened by the fact that we both had serious health issues that appeared in young adulthood, and we realized that our well-being and longevity could not be taken for granted. If we wanted to raise our family and enjoy life for decades to come, we knew we had to make taking care of ourselves and each other a top priority. The silver lining behind a serious medical problem is that it can awaken you to your vulnerability and serve as a call to action to make caring for your body a priority rather than putting everything else first. With the knowledge and modern therapies available today, a proactive, disciplined, and informed person can better deal with whatever medical issues are present.

When James was twenty years old, he was six feet and weighed 154 pounds, as he does now. At the time, he was successfully competing in road-running races and was very fit, or so he thought. In a biochemistry lab, we all drew each other's blood and mixed it with the reagents to measure our own cholesterol levels. James was shocked to find his total cholesterol level above 240. Further testing revealed that his systolic (top) blood pressure was 140 to 160 and his blood sugar was borderline high. When James asked his professors what to do about this, he was less than satisfied with their responses. His family physician dismissed it by telling him he was young and healthy and not to worry about it. But James's intuition told him that his risk profile was a recipe for heart disease at a young age. At that moment, James's career in preventive cardiology began in earnest.

In medical school, we receive embarrassingly little formal training on nutrition and human health. Furthermore, the sanctioned diets from the medical establishment have traditionally been so ineffective in improving health or promoting weight loss that most physicians now harbor a cynical view of the therapeutic value of nutrition. In the 1980s, the diet that was mistakenly touted as the ideal was a very low-fat, low-protein diet that called for eating about 80 percent of calories from carbohydrates. This is the basis of the Pritikin, Ornish, and traditional AHA diets, and they all include white rice, plain baked potatoes, white bagels, orange juice, etc. When James tried such diets, his triglycerides and blood sugar did not go down; in fact, they went up. The cholesterol went down modestly, but the protective HDL cholesterol went down even more and his energy and stamina were not quite what they used to be. Eventually James realized that not all fats were bad; some of them are about the best health food you can eat. Today, we must be reminded that not all carbs are bad either. Fruits and vegetables are the most nutritious components of your diet; it's the processed carbs that should be avoided. As James transitioned to the Forever Young diet, he noticed profound improvements in all of his risk factors. His blood pressure now runs under 115/65, his fasting blood sugar is under 90, his HDL is 60, and his total cholesterol (with the help of a low-dose statin) is under 140.

At age twenty-seven, while six months pregnant with our first child, Joan was diagnosed with metastatic cancer. After she discovered this potentially lethal problem, her attitude immediately changed from one of shock and fear to optimism and resolve. She promised herself that she would do everything in her power to be around to raise her son. We sought out the best medical care, and she courageously endured the surgeries and radiation. Joan's focus on nutrition and fitness was intensified by the experience. She also felt firsthand the healing power of a strong faith, optimism, and a loving, supportive network of family and friends.

Today, Joan is passionately engaged in her nutrition counseling. She often speaks to schools, teams, or families, and women's or men's groups. She has decided this is her community service and donates all of her earnings to charities. Joan calculated that if our youngest child, Caroline, has her last baby at the age she and her mother did, we are going to be in our eighties when our last grandchild is born. She is determined to see that grandchild graduate from high school—which means we will have to hold on until we are about 100. Given that goal and our own health issues, we have a strong personal motivation for making sure the Forever Young program works. We have decided that while it would be nice to live to 100, the real driving force behind our plan is the desire to stay in the prime of our lives—for the rest of our lives. The goal is to thrive, not just survive, and this is now a possibility, thanks to the remarkable advances in knowledge, science, and technology that are included in this program.

Of course, in reality you cannot just read this book and will yourself younger and thinner. An open-minded, optimistic, and adventurous outlook will certainly help you to feel more youthful, but if you really want to turn back the clock you must invest time and energy in the right diet and lifestyle. You may also need to take a few supplements, and depending on your genes and age, one or two prescription medications. We will cover the specifics of the antiaging regimen in later chapters, but the effects that you achieve will be proportional to the time and effort you devote to the cause. Listen to your body and pay attention to what makes you thrive and what depletes your energy. Nobody is perfect, and we all have our health issues. Make sure you know what yours are so you can address them before they damage or even end your life. A recent Harris poll showed that the average American is more likely to know the mileage on his car than his blood pressure. Your car can be replaced—your brain can't. There is no more important priority than keeping your mind and body vigorous and strong.

Carried on the Wings of Hope and Optimism

Deep within you lying dormant are powers that would astonish you—powers beyond anything you have dreamed of possessing. These forces are capable of revolutionizing your life if you discover how to tap into them, and hope is one of the keys to harnessing these inner powers.

A simple and highly reproducible scientific experiment done many years ago dramatically highlights the power of hope. If you place a healthy mouse in a bucket of water it will be able to swim continuously for about thirty minutes before it falters from exhaustion and drowns. However, if you rescue the mouse just as it gives up and slips under the surface and then repeat this cruel experiment again the next day or the next month, that same mouse will now swim for hours, bolstered by hope of another rescue before it drowns.

In every aspect of your life it is better to hope than to despair. Doubt, fear, and despair will drag you down and make you feel old and tired; hope, confidence, and faith will keep you young and strong. James's favorite medical school graduation gift was a worn black leather bag, about the size of an average purse, that once belonged to his great-grandfather Dr. Henry O'Keefe—a pioneer physician who practiced on the North Dakota prairie over 100 years ago. He carried with him something that was more important than the ineffective potions and herbs in that black bag—a promise of hope. Back then "bedside manner" was perhaps the most important measure of a physician because his or her ability to instill a sense of hope and optimism accounted for most of his healing powers. Keep in mind that in those days, people had more confidence in their physician's healing abilities than most of our patients have in doctors today, despite modern medicine's vast array of powerful and effective drugs, surgeries, and high-tech devices.

Joan's ninety-one-year-old mother gets up every morning at five a.m., goes outside to get the paper, and comes back in to declare, "What a glorious morning." A fascinating study in the Mayo Clinic Proceedings in 2002 showed that optimism translates into better health. This trial classified people as optimists, pessimists, or somewhere in between on the basis of a personality inventory taken when they were young adults in the 1960s. The study found that the optimists had a 50 percent lower risk of early death compared to the pessimists during the subsequent thirty years. Harvard researcher Dr. Laura Kubzansky published a study entitled "Is the Glass Half Empty or Half Full?" The paper showed that optimists developed fewer health problems as they aged—less pain, fewer limitations, and higher energy levels. To be sure, optimism and hope are powerful healers.

A famous study followed 180 nuns from the Sisters of Notre Dame Convent in Mankato, Minnesota, from age twenty until old age. Among the notable findings were the enduring positive effects of optimism. Compared to nuns who expressed a more negative outlook in their youth, the nuns who had the most positive attitudes—at ages twenty to twenty-two in handwritten autobiographies—were two and a half times more likely to be alive and healthy well into old age.

Hope springs eternal. Of all the forces that can empower you to change your world, hope may be the most important. It can give you a sense of control and motivate you to do whatever needs to be done. James has witnessed hope's powerful effect on patients with a variety of problems, including high blood pressure, type 2 diabetes, and depression. Every day he sees patients who manage to overcome the powerful nicotine addiction of tobacco by simply deciding to take control of their lives. You probably already know what you need to do to lose that extra weight and regain your fitness, but lasting success will require commitment and perseverance on your part. In order to stick with the plan, you will need optimism and faith in yourself.

You will be on the road to success the moment you start looking within for solutions to your problems. We have learned never to underestimate a person's ability to change his or her life for the better. Believe that you can make it happen, and you just may. How high would you climb if you knew you could not fall? To win out in the end, your desire for success must outweigh your fear of failure. Hope can inspire you with the confidence necessary to make these changes, so cherish your hopes and hold tightly to your dreams. March boldly to the drumbeat that only you can hear.

The price for a cynical, pessimistic attitude is having to live in a hostile and lonely world filled with doubt and worry. My mother used to tell me, "If you don't have something nice to say, at least try to be vague." When you strive to see the best in people and trust that the world is unfolding as it should, life seems easier and happier. Your outlook on life is not an immutable genetically predetermined trait. A more hopeful, trusting, and optimistic attitude is something you can choose for yourself. You can change your mind and change your life. With that outlook and the Forever Young program on the following pages, you may always raise a glass that is half full rather than half empty.

Soar to a "Blue-Sky" Future: The Importance of Your Routine

Your good health is not a gift or a matter of fate, but rather a habit that is cultivated day by day. Over time what you think, choose, and do is what you become. Your life has a trajectory—it is possible to see where you are headed years and even decades before you arrive there by looking closely at what you are doing today. In particular, the path your health follows is determined much less by your genes than your daily habits. Mundane as it seems, your day-to-day routine largely determines how healthy and happy you will be, how quickly you will age, what diseases you will or won't get, and how long you will live.

Life can be hard, but it will be harder if you are careless with your health. Many people spend their life as though they have another one in the bank on reserve. But being alive is like being on board an aircraft flying through a storm: Once you are aloft, you have no option but to make the best of it. A serious oversight or mistake can leave you spiraling out of control and going down in flames without a second chance. Settling into the right routines will keep you flying smoothly for decades to come.

Most of what you do in your day-to-day life is done in the context of a routine. Your health, vigor, and longevity are dependent upon these habits. A routine that involves healthy habits will maintain the integrity of your biosystem and effectively repel the ravages of time and entropy. But if you develop self-defeating customs, they will drag you into the downward spiral of accelerated aging and disease. The key to making your life the best it can be is to develop the right habits, and break the bad habits.

> "Have you ever noticed that people who spend their money
> on cigarettes, beer, and lottery tickets are always complaining
> about being broke and not feeling well?"
> —UNKNOWN

Habits start simply enough, almost unnoticeably. Sharing a cigarette with a friend at a party, grabbing a can of Coke and a bag of potato chips from the vending machine, scarfing down a doughnut in the midmorning because you skipped breakfast, coming home after a long day at work to a big meal and then spending the entire evening watching television. When we find a pattern that feels good or easy, we tend to repeat it. Soon a groove develops in our lives, and the action is no longer a choice but an automatic response; it becomes the path of least resistance. What may have started as innocent whims can eventually become like chains so strong that sometimes you cannot break them to save your life.

Health and vitality are the by-products of small endeavors, repeated consistently day in and day out. Expecting results without hard work is like trying to harvest where you have not planted. Life rewards actions and ignores excuses. The results you get will be proportional to the time and effort you invest into your nutrition and lifestyle. And, unfair as it may seem, with each passing birthday you will have to work a little harder to stay vigorous and youthful.

Habits to Help You Fly Above the Fray

Good habits are as easy to develop as bad ones. Your natural predisposition to develop rituals can be harnessed in a positive sense to "vaccinate" yourself against illness, disease, and aging. If you are like most people, you brush your teeth in the morning and before going to bed. If you also have been disciplined to floss daily, you will almost certainly have healthy teeth and gums for a lifetime. You don't need to think about whether or not to do your daily oral hygiene, it just happens automatically.

My colleague and mentor Robert Conn, MD, likes to say, "If you make it your priority to eat for health rather than taste, you will develop a healthy taste." When that happens, good nutrition becomes second nature and you will just naturally choose the right foods and beverages. Billions of people from cultures around the globe can attest to the fact that green tea can be habit-forming. And it's not for nothing that they call it happy hour—a drink or two before dinner is a routine that can bring relaxation with improved health as an unintended benefit (as long as you limit your "happiness" to not more than two drinks per day). Daily exercise will happen effortlessly if you can find activities that feel more like play and less like work. And sure, sex counts as exercise too, but you will need to find a few other fun activities that get your heart rate up as well.

Our good friend Tom Medlock has a graduate degree from Harvard University and now teaches and coaches at Pembroke Hill High School in Kansas City, Missouri. He wrote to his students in their school paper: *"In cross-country running we practice a lot; we have rituals we repeat many times. They make us stronger, faster, better, more than we were yesterday. The quality of your life practices (routines) factor greatly into what quality of life you have. Do you practice compassion for others? Do you practice self-discipline? Is there a general pattern of giving things your best? Repeat, repeat, repeat, repeat, and you become. But surely repeats are not the purpose of cross country or life. On our team we have a saying: We don't train to train, we train to race. Likewise in life: We don't practice to practice, we practice to fly."*

Rethinking Your Priorities

Bringing balance back to your life is a real key to health and happiness. Living in the twenty-first-century American culture seems to promote an unbalanced life: too much work and not enough play, excessive calories and not enough natural fresh foods, too much stress and not enough fun, and too much TV and too little exercise, too much rushing around—insufficient restful sleep, too much material-ism and too little spirituality. As Dr. Phil would ask, "Is it workin' for ya?" We can tell you that it doesn't work for us. One of the best ways to avoid getting swept away in the tide of the often self-defeating modern lifestyle is to live by the mantra: "Good Things First."

Get in the habit of prioritizing the things that will make your life better in the long run: exercise, eating breakfast each morning, good food and healthy bever-ages, time to play, plenty of rest and relaxation, and a chance to make meaningful connections. When you make it a priority to eat and drink all the good first things first, you will find that you aren't constantly hungry. This makes it easier to resist the junk food temptations that surround you each day.

When you sit down in front of the TV you need to ask yourself, "Have I gotten my exercise today?" If the answer is no, get up and go. At first this may seem uncomfortable, but soon you will feel your energy level improve dramatically, and after a few weeks of daily exercise you will find yourself raring to go. A routine of thirty to sixty minutes of exercise daily will turbo-charge your energy level like nothing else can.

Changing a long-standing habit can be a difficult task. Sometimes a health problem such as a diagnosis of diabetes or high blood pressure, or even a heart attack can be a wake-up call. A reminder of your vulnerability can spur you to make changes in your life that can dramatically improve your future health and longevity. Instead of wasting your precious time and energy worrying about the future or ruminating about the past, focus on what you can do to make you life bet-ter today. You can be truly alive in only one instant—the present moment. The future has not yet arrived, the past is already history. The surest way to take care of the future is to take care of the present and make each moment count.

In James's case he has turned a potentially addictive personality into a positive health habit. He has been "addicted" to exercise from the time he was a small child.

He can remember when, as a college sophomore—after about two decades of having exercise as a mandatory part of his life—it became clear that it was time to give up on organized varsity athletics. However, he made a promise that he would continue to exercise every day, because he knew deep down that this is one of his best coping mechanisms—a crutch that keeps him happy and healthy.

Luck Favors the Prepared

Your life is the product of your choices, actions, thoughts, and words. When you integrate meaningful positive habits into your day-to-day routine, you will flourish and thrive. If you can make these practices a priority in your life and incorporate them into your routine, your excess body fat will melt away and your overall health and well-being will improve. Specific rituals can revolutionize your life and put you on a trajectory toward longevity with energy, health, and vigor. Believe in yourself, make a plan, and begin.

Fourteen Rituals for Longevity That Will Change the Trajectory of Your Life

1. Smile. Think positive. Be optimistic and enthusiastic. You will discover that if you love life, life will love you back.
2. Eat until you are only 80 percent full, and then stop. This is a tradition of the people of Okinawa, the society with the best longevity in the world.
3. Know your numbers. Keep the following levels in the optimal ranges: your blood pressure (under 130/85), cholesterol (under 180), weight (BMI 18 to 25), and sugar (less than 100). Find a doctor you can relate to and trust and see him or her once a year.
4. Try to sleep six to eight and a half hours nightly.
5. Practice good oral hygiene: brush twice and floss once daily.
6. Exercise thirty to sixty minutes every day—if possible.
7. Limit television viewing to not more than two hours daily. Choose shows that make you laugh, make you happy, or enrich your life. Watch TV only after you have gotten your exercise for the day. Or kill two birds with one stone by lifting weights, working out on the treadmill, or doing yoga while viewing television. Even making a meal or folding laundry is better than just sitting on the couch.

8. Get at least fifteen to thirty minutes of fresh air daily.

9. Try to spend at least a few minutes every day in quiet reflection, whether in the form of prayer, meditation, yoga, or relaxation breathing, etc.

10. It's not all about you. Connect with your community and your world. Feel the energy flow into your existence when you make a positive difference in the network of life around you. The universal law of life is that you will only get what you give. If you want a long vigorous life full of health, love, and happiness, it helps to have a generous and caring attitude.

11. Eat fresh natural foods and take time for breakfast each morning. Avoid processed foods, especially anything with hydrogenated polyunsaturated fats (trans fats) or high fructose corn syrup.

12. Include lean protein in your diet three times per day. Consider adding whey protein, one scoop in water or skim milk, for your morning protein source.

13. Each day take three omega-3 (fish oil) capsules (it's OK to take them all at one meal) and a multivitamin.

14. Give up tobacco permanently. Nothing else has the power to improve your health and longevity like stopping smoking for good. Quit making excuses—the nicotine addiction is only brainwashing your mind. Once you have beaten this deadly habit, you will look back and wonder why it took you so long to break free of this ball and chain.

2

THE BEST
OF BOTH WORLDS

Our ancient hunter-gatherer ancestors were sinewy, lean, fit, and vigorous. Although most of our present-day illnesses, including obesity, diabetes, coronary disease, cancer, osteoporosis, depression, and Alzheimer's disease were rare, our ancestors' lives were typically harsh and often violent with a life expectancy of only thirty to forty years. However, those who were clever, hardy, and lucky enough to avoid an early death from infection, childbirth, exposure to the elements, traumatic injuries, parasites, starvation, war, and a host of other potential threats lived into old age with a blood pressure of 110/70, a cholesterol level of about 125, an able body, and a sharp intellect. Life expectancy has doubled today, but most people spend the second half of their lives with a quality of life that is not ideal. No, you don't have to worry about being mauled by a bear or freezing to death in a blizzard, but by the time you reach age forty, you might need prescription medications to compensate for being overweight, achy, depressed, debilitated, or hypertensive. This is no way to live. We like to think of life as a wonderful adventure that you need to train for to fully appreciate all of its beauty and opportunity.

Now it's possible for you not only to have the strength and fitness of your ancestors by living the lifestyle and eating the diet for which you were designed, but also to have the best of modern-day medical technology, such as medications that bring your cholesterol and blood pressure down to the levels that confer longevity, regardless of your genes.

Back to the Future: Becoming a Twenty-first-Century Hunter-Gatherer

You might recall the movie *Jurassic Park,* where dinosaurs were brought back to life by salvaging intact DNA strands from fossils and cloning them. The science of genetics is progressing rapidly, and this may not be such a stretch anymore. If we found a Stone Age human frozen in a glacier 10,000 years ago, extracted intact DNA, and cloned and raised him now, he would pass the subway test. That is, you would not notice anything unusual about him if you sat next to each other and struck up a conversation on a subway train. Our caveman clone would crave sweets and fats, just like you and I do. He would have a tendency to avoid unnecessary physical exertion just like the average sedentary modern American, and subsist on our contemporary synthetic diet. He would also probably become depressed, hypertensive, osteoporotic, obese, and eventually develop heart disease and maybe even cancer. The truth is, our human genome has changed less than 0.03 percent over the past 40,000 years.

Like all living organisms, humans are slaves to their genes. These were selected over thousands of years allowing us to thrive in our natural environment by eating wild game, fish, nuts, berries, fruits, and vegetables, drinking water, and staying very fit while we hunted and gathered nature's bounty. You were designed to use these foods not just for their calories, but also for the multitude of antiaging and disease-fighting nutrients they contain. Modern food manufacturers strip away these essential nutrients, leaving only empty calories in the form of sugar, starch, and fat, and then add unnatural chemicals like high fructose corn syrup, hydrogenated oils (trans fats), preservatives, and artificial colors. The end results are usually deliciously tempting, convenient treats that are then heavily marketed making them almost irresistible.

The caveman 10,000 years ago would much rather have gulped down a cheeseburger, fries, and a Coke than risked his life tracking and killing an untamed antelope, digging up wild onions, or climbing a tree to pick fruit. Since he did not have that choice, he stayed strong, lean, and vigorous eating only natural whole foods. Today, you can eat essentially the same foods and reap the same health benefits, but you will have to learn what it is that you are designed to eat and develop the self-discipline to voluntarily follow this program.

Until relatively recently, people ate only wild, unprocessed "real" food hunted and gathered from nature. They ate a diet high in lean protein, omega-3 and monounsaturated fats, fiber, vitamins and minerals, and antioxidants. These ancestors were healthy, fit, strong, and free from obesity and related diseases—like cardiovascular disease and high blood pressure—that are the norm in our modern world. Their bones and teeth were strong and healthy during their entire lives, and cancer was a rare illness.

Today, most of us live in mechanized, urban settings leading sedentary lifestyles and eating a diet of processed synthetic food. As a result, two-thirds of us are overweight or obese, 90 percent of us develop high blood pressure, and 40 percent die from cardiovascular disease. Type 2 diabetes, a rare disease a few generations ago, is now a full-fledged epidemic, with a 40 percent increase in the past decade alone.

Despite the astounding advances in drugs and biomedical technology, the epidemic of obesity continues to increase 1 percent per year. The number of very obese people is rising faster than any other group of overweight Americans, with a three-fold rise in the past fourteen years. So do not feel persecuted—your struggle to control your weight is not your fault—you are living in an environment that is alien to your genetic identity.

Socially we are the people of a highly advanced technological civilization, but from a genetic perspective, we remain citizens of the Paleolithic Era that ended 10,000 years ago. Most of our health problems today result from this mismatch between the world we are designed for and the very different one we live in—we are organisms that are living out of context. Millions of years of natural selection ensured that our bodies and minds were genetically adapted to thrive while hunting and gathering on the grasslands of the plains, but when it comes to a sedentary lifestyle of automobiles, couches, televisions, computers, and junk food, we are like fish out of water.

Radically changing our diet and lifestyle hasn't altered our genetic identity any more than dying brown hair blond increases the chances that one's offspring will be blond. You might like to kid yourself into thinking that you will stay healthy in living your fast-food, high-stress sedentary lifestyle because it's all you have ever known. In reality, your chances of thriving while drinking colas and eating glazed doughnuts and watching TV for most of your waking hours are no better than for a cactus trying to grow in a rain forest. Your ancient genetic blueprint compels you to remain faithful to your true nature or degenerate into poor health and spiritual malaise.

Compared to the modern diet you are eating today our ancestor's diet contained two to three times more fiber, six times more omega-3 fats, two times more monounsaturated fat, and 70 percent less saturated fat. Protein intake was three times higher and the potassium intake was fourfold higher, but the sodium intake was only one-sixth of what we consume today. They consumed no refined sugars; *today the average adult eats 150 pounds of sugar per year, and teenagers eat 250 pounds of sugar per year.* Most important, they burned virtually all the calories they consumed and only occasionally, during seasons of abundance, did they have the chance to put on a few pounds of stored fat. The ongoing epidemics of obesity, diabetes, and cardiovascular disease today are in large part due to the striking differences between the diet we were designed to eat and the synthetic age-accelerating calorie-dense—but nutrient-poor—food we are actually eating.

Nine Steps Toward a Hunter-Gatherer's Diet

If you want to be in synch with your genetic heritage, here are the steps you should follow to become a hunter-gatherer.

1. Thrive on the earth's natural bounty. Eat whole, natural, fresh foods; avoid highly processed foods.

2. Consume a diet high in fruits, vegetables, nuts, and berries, and low in refined grains and sugars.

3. Increase consumption of omega-3 fatty acids from fish, fish oil, and plant sources like walnuts, canola oil, greens, soybeans, and flaxseed.

4. Avoid trans fats entirely. Eliminate fried foods, hard margarine, commercial baked goods, and most packaged and processed snack foods. Also limit consumption of fatty meats and high-fat dairy.

5. Increase consumption of lean protein such as skinless poultry, fish, game meats, and whey protein. Eat only lean, fresh cuts of red meat and limit consumption of saturated fats, including fatty, salty processed meats like bacon, sausage, and deli meats.

6. Incorporate olive oil or canola oil into your diet. Avoid corn, safflower, sunflower, and vegetable oils.

7. Choose purified water, tea, nonfat unsweetened dairy or soymilk, and red wine. Avoid soft drinks, fruit juices, high-fat dairy, and sports drinks. Even 100 percent fruit juices are still loaded with too much sugar and should be considered off-limits. However, low-sodium vegetable juices are very nutritious.

8. Use your body as it was designed and programmed over the millennia and engage in daily exercise from a variety of activities that incorporate aerobic and strength training as well as stretching exercises. Outdoor activities are ideal.

9. Develop and maintain relationships that provide social support (e.g., spouse, family, friends, neighbors, community, etc.). Try to also include some activities that involve altruism and nurturing.

We will discuss the importance of many of these nutrition recommendations later in this chapter.

The Fab Four Longevity Factors

Mainstream medicine can prevent disease and improve longevity by prescribing safe medications to control risk factors like high cholesterol and hypertension. Yet this passive pharmaceutical approach to your health is inadequate when used alone to protect against aging and premature death. You will also need to make it a priority to follow a healthful lifestyle that can help to prevent chronic disease in the first place.

Literally tens of thousands of scientific studies make it abundantly clear that following the right lifestyle can extend the average person's healthy lifespan a number of years. One of the strongest testimonies to the power of diet and exercise was published September 23, 2004, in the *Journal of the American Medical Association*. This rigorously conducted study of 2,339 men and women from several European countries concluded that adopting the following Fab Four simple lifestyle habits *will cut the risk of death during a ten-year period by about 65 percent*:

1. Regular physical activity (defined as at least thirty minutes exercise per day) conferred a 37 percent decreased risk of death (from any cause).

2. Not smoking tobacco was associated with a 35 percent lower risk.

3. Consuming a Mediterranean diet lowered the mortality risk by 23 percent.

4. Regular consumption of low to moderate amounts of alcohol was associated with a 22 percent lower risk.

These habits reduced mortality rates for both heart disease and cancer to a similar degree. *Following all four of these diet/lifestyle recommendations dropped the risk of dying during the study period by two-thirds compared to practicing one or none of the Fab Four healthy habits.* It sounds easy enough, but the July/August 2005 issue of *AARP: The Magazine* reported that 97 percent of U.S. adults don't follow all four of these rules for healthy living.

Eat Like the Mediterranean People

Last summer Joan and I took our family to La Ciotat, a small village on the Mediterranean coast in southern France—the home of the real Mediterranean diet. We found this to be the most delicious and healthiest cuisine we have ever experienced and were very inspired by how the French people eat and live. We also noticed that the women of all ages tended to have small, sexy waists, and smooth and beautiful complexions despite the fact that these people were not fitness buffs. There was one gym in town, and it was used only for playing squash. They didn't get their toned abs from doing hundreds of sit-ups daily or taking some weight-loss supplement. No, the beautiful flat tummies with the pierced belly buttons are the by-product of an active lifestyle and a diet that keeps their hormones in the healthy youthful ranges. In contrast, the average tubby American continues his or her futile struggle with the "Ab-blaster" machine and fad diets, while eating synthetic foods loaded with trans fats and high fructose corn syrup and spending most of the day sitting in front of a TV or computer screen.

In her best-selling book French Women Don't Get Fat *Mireille Guiliano states that "The French know you can eat everything; the trick is balancing it and eating small portions. We don't obsess about food—we're friends with it." Other features of the Mediterranean diet and lifestyle include:*

> *Drink water throughout the day.*
>
> *Eat three meals per day, no snacks.*
>
> *Avoid processed foods.*
>
> *Do not eat standing up, on the run, or in front of the TV or computer screen.*
>
> *Enjoy wine regularly but not more than a glass or two.*
>
> *Enjoy dark chocolate in moderation.*
>
> *Move your body. Climb the stairs, walk everywhere you can.*

Taken in composite, scientific studies relating to diet show that only four dietary interventions consistently improve overall health: 1) cut daily caloric intake; 2) add fresh, natural, whole plant foods like vegetables, fruits, berries, and nuts; 3) increase omega-3 fats, especially in the form of a fish oil supplement; 4) substitute healthy mono and polyunsaturated oils from plants such as nuts, olive oil, avocados, and soybeans for unhealthy saturated fats found in animals and high-fat dairy, and the toxic trans fats in deep-fried foods, margarines, processed snack foods, and commercial baked goods. All four of these principles are part of the traditional Mediterranean diet.

Americans equate pasta and pizza with a Mediterranean diet. In fact, the French do eat some of these foods and French bread too—but the portion sizes of these starches are small. The striking difference in their diet, however, is the amount of fresh produce and fish that they eat. Each morning the market in La Ciotat was crowded with people, all filling their carts with a remarkable variety of delicious fresh vegetables and fruits. The largest line in the store was at the fish counter, where you could choose from over thirty different varieties of fresh fish and shellfish. They prepare their food with olive oil, and eat minimal fried foods and are not big on packaged processed foods. Although the Mediterraneans love their coffee, tea, red wine, cheese, milk, and even cigarettes, their rate of heart disease is much lower than in America.

Today, you can eat the Mediterranean diet anywhere, anytime. Your choices may be a bit more limited, but fresh produce, lean meat, and fish are almost always available. Imagine yourself a twenty-first-century hunter-gatherer bringing home fresh produce, nuts, and fresh meat or fish every other day or so. Just like the townspeople of La Ciotat, Joan goes to the local supermarket about every second day, but spends just about twelve minutes there picking up fresh items. We also try to keep our home stocked with staples like nuts, frozen mixed berries, bottled water, sparkling water, wine, skim milk, soymilk, cholesterol-free or omega-3 enriched eggs, frozen seafood, chicken breasts, and dark chocolate.

Healthy Fats

The primitive human diet was higher in good fats like omega-3 fats and monounsaturated fats but lower in the bad fats—trans fats and saturated fats—than our modern diet. The omega-3 and monounsaturated fats are abundant in fish, nuts, and game meats. In the winter months when fruits and vegetables were not available, our ancestors lived exclusively on foods like nuts and lean meat from wild game. These foods have been shown to lower risks of diabetes, cardiovascular disease, sudden death, and obesity.

Some modern foods like olive oil and dark chocolate are other sources of healthy fats and antioxidants. Adding the omega-3 and monounsaturated fats to your diet can revitalize the way you feel and look. These good fats help to keep your skin smooth and supple, your brain youthful, your mood upbeat, and your heart and arteries clean, soft, and pliable. Most Americans are deficient in these beneficial fats and are overwhelmed with saturated and trans fats—unnatural fats that cause your tissues to become rigid and inflamed and ultimately lead to accelerated aging and disease.

The fat in avocados is the same heart-healthy version found in olive oil. Avocados are also rich in fiber and beta-sitosterol (natural cholesterol-lowering phytonutrients), and vitamins E, C, B$_6$, and riboflavin. In order to efficiently absorb lutein, beta-carotene, and other disease-fighting antiaging carotenoids, you must eat them with some healthy fat. A recent study by Steven Schwartz, PhD, found that avocado acts as a nutrient booster. Study subjects who ate avocado with their spinach salad absorbed thirteen and one-half times more beta-carotene and four times more lutein than those who ate the salad without avocado.

Chocolate as Health Food?

Dark chocolate is a rich source of antioxidants, and the fat present in this treat is metabolically neutral, like olive oil. This is the only candy with any nutritional value and can be allowed in very small quantities after the weight loss (induction) phase of the Forever Young diet.

A study of twenty patients with mild high blood pressure who were treated with chocolate was published in the July 2005 issue of the journal *Hypertension*. This study reported that 100 grams (about three ounces) of dark chocolate daily for three weeks caused a twelve-point reduction in their systolic (top) blood pressure with a 13 percent drop in the bad cholesterol level. White chocolate showed no benefit in this study. Additionally, dark chocolate improved the health of the blood vessels by making the arteries more relaxed and responsive. Finally, measurement of insulin sensitivity (predisposition to diabetes) was also improved in the patients who received the dark chocolate, but not in patients who received the white chocolate. These benefits were attributed to the presence of high levels of beneficial antiaging flavonoids in dark chocolate.

The type of chocolate makes all the difference. Milk chocolate is high in sugar and milk fat and low in antioxidants, and it will expand your waistline, not your arteries. White chocolate is not chocolate at all, and the instant cocoa mixes you find at the supermarket contain only low levels of antioxidants and may include saturated fats from palm oil. Cheaper brands of chocolate are mostly sugar and often substitute toxic hydrogenated vegetable oils for cocoa butter.

If you want health-food grade chocolate, look for a product that is at least 60 percent cocoa solids by weight. The first ingredient in a high-quality chocolate bar should be cocoa solids, cocoa mass, cocoa, cacao, cocoa butter, or chocolate liquor. Baking chocolate is 100 percent cocoa and is practically inedible, and most people find chocolate bars with greater than 85 percent cocoa too bitter to enjoy. We prefer chocolate that is 70 to 75 percent cocoa and find that a small chunk (or square) can be savored for a few minutes. Good-quality dark chocolate is high in calories, so you have to limit yourself to not more than about twenty grams (two-thirds of an ounce or 100 calories) daily. Dark chocolate–covered nuts are a highly nutritious (but high-calorie) treat; limit yourself to not more than about ten per serving.

Tip: *Make a delicious healthy dessert by cutting up fresh fruits such as strawberries, apples, peaches, or pears and mixing together with small squares of a high-quality chocolate bar. Serve with hot tea or coffee, and you will have a pleasurable treat that qualifies as health food.*

Trans Fats: The Deadliest (and Best-Tasting) Food on the Planet

The unhealthiest food or food ingredient on the planet is trans fat. In July 2002, the National Academy of Science studied the research on these dangerous substances and came to the conclusion that "the only safe intake of trans fats is zero." These fats have been banished from the food supply in Holland and should be banned (but are not) in America as well. Trans fats, also known as hydrogenated or partially hydrogenated fats, are unnatural and toxic and will ruin your health if consumed frequently. Our hunter-gatherer ancestors ate virtually none of these.

Hydrogenated fats remain the darlings of the processed food industry. The most common sources of trans fats in today's diet are deep-fried foods, especially French fries, commercial baked goods (doughnuts, cookies, cakes, croissants, etc.), margarines, and snack foods such as crackers and chips. Trans fats usually taste delicious, and manufacturers love their long shelf life. Your system will preferentially incorporate these unnatural fats into your cell membranes to the exclusion of healthy fats such as omega-3 oils. A diet high in trans fats results in stiffening of the membranes, eventually transforming supple, healthy organs into waxy, rigid, and dysfunctional tissues. On average, we consume only 2 percent of our calories in the form of trans fats. However, if we eliminated these from our diet altogether, the rate of heart attack and coronary death would drop by about 50 percent. Trans fats also accelerate aging and predispose us to many other serious diseases, such as cancer, diabetes, and dementia. Fortunately, food manufacturers must list trans fat content, so read the labels and avoid all foods that contain trans fats. Also, never eat deep-fried foods or commercial baked goods.

Go Nuts

Health nuts like us are crazy about nuts these days, and for good reasons. Our enthusiasm is fueled by a steady stream of impressive scientific studies showing that nuts seem to protect against heart attack, sudden death, obesity, diabetes, and high cholesterol. They are a unique natural food loaded with protein, healthy fats, vegetable protein, vitamin E (including the most important form of this nutrient—gamma tocopherol), folate, fiber, potassium, magnesium, and a host of nutrients and antioxidants like tannins and polyphenols. Humans are designed to have nuts in their diet, and studies show that moderate nut consumption is linked to better health. Unsalted or low-sodium tree nuts are best, but even peanuts are okay. Just make sure they are fresh; aflatoxin, a mold that grows on old and stale peanuts, is a potent carcinogen.

A one- to two-ounce (one-quarter of a cup) serving of nuts is an ideal snack. We encourage people to eat them on a daily basis. Tree nuts (walnuts, pecans, Brazil nuts, almonds, hazelnuts, etc.) are a valuable source of omega-3 fat similar to that found in oily fish (such as salmon, trout, tuna, sea bass). In studies this plant-based form of omega-3, alpha-linolenic acid, has been shown to reduce LDL (bad) cholesterol and also cool the fires of inflammation as measured by C-reactive protein (CRP) levels. These omega-3 fats are used by the body to make DHA—the fatty acid that is incorporated into the cell walls of tissues in the heart, blood vessels, and brain to help keep these organs soft, supple, and youthful.

Peanut butter is a wonderful food that is quick, scrumptious, and healthy. A slice of hearty, dense, whole-grain bread smeared with a natural peanut butter spread is a delicious part of a meal or snack. It is loaded with metabolically neutral monounsaturated fat, so it will not raise your cholesterol or blood pressure. This is the kind of food that keeps you satiated for hours and is convenient and versatile. You can eat it on raw vegetables like celery and carrots, or fruits like apples and bananas. Look for the natural peanut butter brands to make sure that the tasty stuff getting stuck to the roof of your mouth contains no hydrogenated or partially hydrogenated fats.

Tip: *Store natural peanut butter upside down in your refrigerator. This will allow the oil that separates out to rise to the bottom of the jar. When you first take it out and use it, you will want to stir the peanut butter well but you won't have to deal with a layer of oil on the top.*

It has been estimated that eating one ounce of nuts daily will reduce your risk of fatal coronary heart disease by 45 percent when substituted for saturated fat (fatty meats like sausage or full-fat dairy products) and about 30 percent when substituted for processed carbohydrate (snack foods high in sugar or starch). It is essential to substitute nuts for other snacks to reap their full health benefits. Interestingly, the natural human diet has always included nuts, which provide a good source of energy and nutrition. During the scarcity of a barren winter, our ancestors relied on them as a valuable source of calories. Nuts and seeds nurture developing life and contain many of the nutrients essential for health.

Although nuts contain a high proportion of fat (up to 80 percent of calories), it's good fat. Tree nuts are actually low in saturated fat and contain no cholesterol. Peanuts, which are technically legumes rather than nuts, have a slightly higher proportion of saturated fat, but are still OK. However, avoid the heavily salted and honey roasted varieties since these are high in both salt and sugar. Even though nuts are high in calories, studies show that adding them to the diet does not usually cause weight gain. In contrast, people who eat nuts regularly tend to be less prone to obesity than those who do not eat them. Some evidence indicates that people who eat large amounts of nuts do not absorb some of the fat, accounting for some of the protection against obesity that nuts provide. The Forever Young diet encourages moderate consumption of nuts along with fruits, vegetables, beans, and other healthy plant-based foods.

There are a number of studies to support the fact that eating nuts can prevent heart disease. The most convincing evidence comes from several large population studies. The first of these was the Seventh-Day Adventist Health Study, involving over 31,000 people. Researchers found that those who reported eating nuts more than four times per week had a 50 percent lower risk of coronary heart disease compared to those who rarely ate nuts. Virtually identical results were seen in a study of 86,000 women followed for fourteen years. The women who ate nuts frequently decreased their risk of heart disease by 50 percent compared to those who did not. When the researchers controlled for multiple risk factors like smoking, cholesterol, exercise, and diet, the frequent nut eaters still had a 35 percent lower risk.

Mixed Nuts: The Best Choice

When people ask us what nut is best, we usually answer, mixed nuts. Variety in natural whole foods is ideal, and eating a handful of mixed nuts gives you a real spectrum of healthy nutrients. Walnuts are rich in the plant-based omega-3 fats that help to curb cravings, among other benefits. Just one or two Brazil nuts will provide as much selenium as an expensive supplement; pistachios are uniquely high in lutein and zeaxanthin to keep your eyes and heart healthy; almonds are rich in vitamin E and folic acid. Among nuts, pecans are highest in antioxidants, and many nuts, including peanuts, walnuts, almonds, hazelnuts, and macadamia nuts, are high in plant sterols such as campesterol and beta-sitosterol that can lower cholesterol levels. Try to look for unsalted or lightly salted mixed nuts.

Evidence therefore suggests that eating nuts may help reduce the risk of heart disease, diabetes, and maybe even obesity. The mechanism for this protection is not fully understood, but it probably relates to reductions in cholesterol, triglycerides, and sugar, as well as antioxidant effects. Nuts are high in calories, so you have to eat them in moderation. Joan advises people to have one handful daily, but reminds them with a smile that they must be able to close their fists around their nuts to make it a legitimate serving size. If only salted nuts are available, rinse them under running water to wash the salt off. Fresh nuts in the shell are a great treat if you have the time, and having to shell each one makes it easier to keep your intake moderate. Buy small quantities that you can use within a month or so and store them in the refrigerator or freezer to keep them fresh. Avoid grinding your own peanut or almond butter at the health food store—this process exposes the nuts to excessive oxygen, which accelerates oxidation of the fats and leads to rancidity. Nuts make a great snack to keep handy at work as an alternative to the junk food in the vending machines. If you're looking for a delicious, convenient, and healthy snack, fresh, natural nuts are at the top of the list.

Fiber Is Your Friend

Your body is designed to process more than forty grams of fiber a day. The average American eats less than a third of this amount (twelve grams per day), which is one of the reasons why constipation, esophageal reflux (heartburn), hemorrhoids, diabetes, diverticulosis, and colon cancer are common ailments in our population. We recommend that you shoot for twenty-five to forty grams of fiber daily. To achieve this, you will have to make an effort to eat at least nine servings (four and one-half cups) of fruits and vegetables daily and to also eat nuts, whole grains, and legumes on a daily basis. Citrus fruits (especially grapefruits), berries, plums, and prunes are especially rich sources of fiber. Read the label on bread and find one that provides four or even five grams of fiber with each slice. Some brands also have added calcium, vitamin D, and folic acid, but most contain high fructose corn syrup, which is one reason why we don't recommend that you eat more than one or two slices daily.

Billions of dollars are spent each year on powerful drugs that shut down the natural acid-producing capability of the stomach in an attempt to reduce heartburn and gastroesophageal reflux. Most of these people's lifelong problems with reflux could be cured by simply consuming a high-fiber, high-water diet and eliminating processed and salty foods. A high-fiber diet will not just help you lose weight but will also prevent constipation, slightly lower blood pressure and cholesterol, and decrease your risks of heart disease and colon cancer.

A recent study from Tufts University found that a high-fiber diet was effective in preventing obesity. The researchers evaluated 459 adults and found that people who frequently consumed fruit, legumes, whole grains, and reduced-fat dairy products had waists that were on average two inches smaller than those who ate fewer of these foods. Lead author P. K. Newby, PhD, attributed the lower level of abdominal fat in part to the high-fiber content of most of these foods.

You can obtain about sixteen grams of fiber by eating a single cup of kidney beans, which are easily added to salads, soups, or stews. Beans are loaded with the same antiaging, disease-preventing phytonutrients found in red wine, berries, and tea. Among the varieties of beans, red kidney beans and black beans are highest in these beneficial plant-based compounds followed (in decreasing order) by small red beans, pinto, brown, yellow, and white beans. One-half cup of red kidney beans or black beans has the same antioxidant content as two glasses of red wine.

What Are You Drinking?

The beverages you choose to drink on a daily basis play a major role in your long-term health. If you routinely gulp down sugared sodas as your default beverage choice, you will be more likely to have weight problems, diabetes, a bad complexion, and even cardiovascular disease. Better choices include clean pure water, green or even black tea, coffee in moderation, nonfat milk, and soymilk. Try to avoid sodas, diet sodas, sports drinks, juices, sugared drinks, and excessive alcohol.

Our ancestors drank water almost exclusively. Studies show that generous water intake may reduce the risks of heart attack and stroke. Aim for at least eight glasses of water per day. Tea, especially green tea, is another healthy beverage that has been linked to lower risks for heart attack, cardiac death, and cancer.

We strongly recommend that you try to consume three or more cups of tea per day along with one or two glasses of nonfat milk or soymilk. Caffeinated coffee is acceptable, but try to keep your total daily intake to not more than two cups.

A recent study out of the Netherlands found that drinking four or more cups of coffee per day raises homocysteine levels, which could theoretically increase risk of cardiovascular disease. You can drink as much green tea as you like, but if you are drinking more than four cups per day, consider using a decaf variety for your afternoon and evening cups of tea. Try to mix about twenty grams of whey protein powder into one of your beverages (best in water, skim milk, or soymilk) during the day. Whey protein is one of the single best foods you can consume (see chapter 3).

The Problem with Vegetarianism

All experts agree that humans are genetically designed to be omnivorous. In fact, the best studies indicate that our ancestors obtained about 50 to 65 percent of their calories from animal sources. Strictly vegetarian diets are difficult to follow and not necessarily associated with better health. Recent studies show that people who eat grains, vegetables, and fruits exclusively are not as healthy as those who include lean protein such as fish and fresh lean red meat in their diet.

In 2002 nobody was too surprised when Dave Thomas, the good-natured founder and spokesperson for Wendy's fast-food chain, died at age sixty-nine of heart disease after enduring heart attacks, coronary bypass surgeries, and other cardiac catastrophes for decades. Of course, the Wendy's organization denied any connection between his heart disease and a lifelong diet of double bacon cheeseburgers and French fries. When Jim Cantalupo, McDonald's CEO and company veteran for three decades, died at age sixty in April 2004 of a heart attack, Charlie Bell took over the reins at the Golden Arches. Bell was also a lifer with McDonald's, and only two weeks after the forty-four-year-old assumed the CEO position, he underwent surgery for colorectal cancer. He died of cancer just nine months later. It doesn't take a high-powered biostatistician to deduce that consuming fast food on a daily basis for decades may qualify as an occupational hazard. To be fair, McDonald's and other fast-food restaurants are only selling what the public wants, and today they also have healthy, fresh, whole, natural food choices like salads, fruit, low-fat yogurt and milk, and bottled water.

A less well-publicized, but much more surprising catastrophe befell Jay Dinshah, the founder and president of the American Vegan Society, which advocates eating no meat, eggs, dairy, fish, or animal products of any kind. Mr. Dinshah was raised in a strictly vegetarian household and followed a vegan diet his entire life. He died at sixty-six of a heart attack despite the fact that he had never tasted a burger during his entire life. Here was a guy who probably boycotted animal crackers just on principle, yet he succumbed to what was supposed to be the scourge of meat-eaters. These untimely deaths in high-profile people highlight what's wrong with the American diet. A fare of unnatural, highly processed, calorie-dense, fast foods like fries, chicken nuggets, and shakes is clearly not what we are designed to eat, but neither is a diet that is devoid of meat, fish, and seafood. *The simple and intuitive biologic truth is that if you eat the food for which your body is genetically adapted, you will thrive. If you don't, you will suffer adverse health consequences.*

Recent studies on vegetarians show little to no survival advantage for this eating style. A trial of 8,000 vegetarians followed for sixteen years showed no difference in mortality rates or risk of heart disease, cancer, and stroke between vegetarians and meat-eaters. In fact, that study showed similar rates for all but two of the top twelve diseases—breast cancer and degenerative brain disorders like Alzheimer's disease that were both *higher* in the vegetarian populations! Shockingly, the vegetarians had twice the risk of developing fatal brain diseases. A study published in the September 2003 issue of the *American Journal of Clinical Nutrition* followed 17,000 vegetarians for ten years. Once again, the vegetarians had the same overall mortality rate as meat-eaters.

Keep in mind that vegetarians as a group have lower rates of obesity, diabetes, colon cancer, high blood pressure, high cholesterol, and appendicitis. Yet, vegetarians may not live longer despite the fact that they consume much less saturated fat and virtually none of carcinogenic compounds found in the overprocessed, overcooked carcinogenic meats that are staples in the modern diet. It would only seem fair that after a life of forgoing the pleasures like filet mignon and grilled salmon, vegetarians would have a little extra time to show for it—but they don't.

Most modern-day vegetarians more appropriately would be labeled "breaditarians." Studies consistently find that even health-conscious vegetarians seldom meet the old recommendation of five or more servings of fresh fruits and vegetables per day. On the Forever Young program we want you to eat at least nine servings of produce per day and still leave room for nuts, meat, fish, dairy, and eggs. Instead of fresh produce, most vegetarians are busily consuming large amounts of processed carbohydrates such as rice, potatoes, white flour, and sugars.

Besides not getting enough high-quality protein, vegetarians usually are deficient in nutrients such as omega-3 fats, vitamin B_{12}, vitamin D, and zinc. That is a recipe for poor brain, nerve, and heart health. DHA and other omega-3 fats are the preferred fats to incorporate into the walls of brain and nerve cells. Deficiency of this crucial fat has been strongly linked to a great many diseases including depression, attention-deficit hyperactivity disorder, Alzheimer's disease, and sudden death. Vitamin B_{12} is also critical for maintaining normal homocysteine levels and healthy nerves and blood vessels. Because we are omnivores by design, we must eat animal foods like fish and seafood, lean poultry and red meat to obtain optimum levels of these critical nutrients. If you choose, however, to follow a strictly vegetarian diet, make sure to take a multivitamin, at least 1000 mg of DHA (an omega-3 fat that can be derived from algae to make it acceptable even for vegans), use two scoops of whey protein per day, and eat lots of vegetables and fruits!

Meat as Health Food

The best science indicates that our ancient ancestors consumed over half of their calories from animal sources. As a young man who virtually grew up outdoors in North Dakota, which looks like a white frozen tundra in winter, I often pondered what the Native Americans were eating when they inhabited this land. They certainly would have scavenged leftover nuts and berries, but these alone would not have been enough to keep them alive and strong through a long harsh winter. In fact, by the time the snowflakes appeared, the tribes were subsisting on meat from the herds of deer, buffalo, and other plentiful game species that lived on the prairie during the winter.

Paradoxically, this meat-based hunter-gatherer diet was associated with excellent overall health, low rates of obesity, and healthy hearts. How could this be? Well, for starters, the animals that they ate typically had only 4 percent saturated fat by weight, yet they were relatively rich in healthy fats like omega-3 oils and monounsaturated fat. Today's meats usually come from grain-fed domestic animals that typically contain 25 to 30 percent fat by weight, much of it in the form of unhealthy saturated fat. So, learn to choose only lean cuts of red meat such as those with the words "round" or "loin" in the name, and trim away any visible fat. Other healthy protein sources include fish, eggs, skinless poultry, nuts, whey protein, and nonfat dairy.

Another major problem associated with many modern meats is an increased cancer risk due to unnatural compounds added during cooking and/or processing. Two studies published in the January 12, 2005, issue of the *Journal of the American Medical Association* found that people who eat red meat frequently (nine or more servings per week) have a 30 to 40 percent increased risk of colon and rectal cancers compared with those who eat little or no red meat. These findings should be kept in perspective: Physical inactivity, obesity, and smoking all appear to increase the risk of colon/rectal cancer to a greater degree than frequently eating red meat. Much of that increased risk can also be avoided if you do not eat charred or overdone red meat and limit your consumption of meat, fish, and poultry that has been fried or grilled until well done. Cured meats such as hot dogs, hams, and luncheon meats are high in nitrosamines, which also are suspected to play a role in cancers, especially of the gastrointestinal tract. Again, the problems are solved if you eat meat in its most natural form—fresh, lean, and not burned or cooked at high temperatures.

Your ideal diet is not low-carb, or low-fat, or vegetarian. Carbohydrates, fats, and animal foods are all essential to optimum health and vitality. Lean fresh meat keeps you strong and healthy; fatty, processed, and overcooked meat causes heart disease and cancer. Carbohydrates from brightly or deeply colored vegetables and fruits, whole grains, and legumes make you energetic and youthful; processed empty carbs like white sugar and white flour make you overweight, diabetic, and depressed. Beneficial oils like omega-3 and extra virgin olive oil prevent aging and disease; toxic fats like saturated and trans fats cause Alzheimer's disease, inflammation, and hardening of the arteries. The key is to choose the natural, fresh versions of the foods you eat.

The Atkins diet devotees are on target when they shun processed carbs like doughnuts and soft drinks, but they do eat too much saturated fat and salt and not enough healthy antioxidants from fruits and vegetables. The vegetarians are on track when they avoid saturated fat, but then they binge on the processed carbs and miss out on essential nutrients like omega-3 fat and vitamin B_{12}, which are readily available only in animal foods. So the solution is to eat like your ancient ancestors and thrive on the fare for which your genes are designed: at least nine servings of vegetables and fruit daily, plenty of fiber including some from whole grains and legumes, lean protein three times daily, lots of water and tea, and plenty of omega-3 fat. This is the diet that will bring out the best in you and give you longevity with vigor.

What Is Good for the Heart Is Good for the Brain

The ramifications of the aging brain are a looming catastrophe for our society as the baby boomers spiral toward a collective generational senior moment. Preserving razor-sharp brain function is critically important to achieving and enjoying longevity with meaning. Keeping your mind forever young requires daily exercise, eating right, and making sure that your cholesterol and blood pressure levels are in the ideal ranges.

The Kaiser Permanente Health System tracked the health of 9,000 people who were in their early forties. This study, published in January 2005, found that people with one or more of the common heart risk factors (high blood pressure, diabetes, high cholesterol, and smoking) were at increased risk for dementia later in life. The well-being of the brain is critically dependent upon healthy blood vessels to supply energy in the form of glucose and oxygen. The beauty of this unified-disease concept is that what we do for our heart also pays off for our brain and memory. In other words, healthier arteries promote clearer thinking. Studies consistently show that interventions to improve heart health such as exercise, omega-3 fats, statins, blood pressure control, aspirin, stress reduction, and a healthy diet are all good for the brain as well.

You are only as young as your brain. A happy, curious, creative, and sharp mind is essential to staying youthful. Medical science has made remarkable progress in recent years regarding nutritional strategies for attaining and preserving optimal brain function, intellect, and mood. Some studies identify dietary factors that reduce the risks of declining cognition and diseases such as Alzheimer's, dementia, and stroke. Others have highlighted foods that improve mood, memory, concentration, and even IQ. Remember to keep these foods in your diet on a daily basis, and you will be more apt to remember everything else, and be joyful and enthused at the same time.

Consume Foods Rich in Omega-3 Fats:
- Fish, seafood, and game meat
- Green leafy vegetables such as purslane, broccoli, cauliflower, spinach, and others
- Pharmaceutical-grade (at least 60 percent DHA + EPA) omega-3 fish oil supplement. Suggested dose is about 1500 to 2000 mg daily. If you buy standard fish oil (which is about 30 percent omega-3 by weight) from a pharmacy or discount center like Costco, you will need to take three to six capsules (1000 mg each) daily.
- Walnuts and flaxseed

Consume Foods High in Vitamin E and Other Tocopherols:
- Nuts (especially tree nuts)
- Canola oil
- Soybean oil
- Wheat germ

Consume Fruits and Vegetables Rich in Antioxidants:
- Blackberries, blueberries, strawberries, raspberries
- Cherries
- Bell peppers (red, green, orange)
- Citrus fruits (oranges, grapefruits, tangerines, lemons, limes)
- Artichokes
- Apples

- Spinach, kale, greens
- Kiwi
- Cantaloupe
- Broccoli, brussels sprouts
- Nectarines
- Carrots
- Dried plums (prunes), not more than five per day

Consume Foods Naturally Rich in Folic Acid:
- Citrus fruits (see above)
- Beans
- Green leafy vegetables (see above)
- Avocados

Haste Makes Waist

Robert Vogel, MD, from the University of Maryland is an expert in vascular biology. He and his colleagues studied the effects of diet on blood vessel function in healthy volunteers before and after a high trans fat, high-calorie, fast-food meal. In the study, blood vessel function deteriorated temporarily after a single meal at McDonald's to the same degree as that noted after smoking two cigarettes. Dr. Vogel jokes that when you take your children over to McDonald's for a Happy Meal of French fries, chicken nuggets, and a cola, you might just as well take them out behind the garage to smoke a couple of cigarettes.

Super-Size Me is an award-winning documentary about the devastating effects of a steady diet of fast food. In the film, a healthy, fit thirty-three-year-old man commits himself to eating three meals a day for thirty consecutive days at McDonald's. If he is asked, "Want to supersize that?" he is obligated to do so, and he must finish all of the food at each meal. In the span of the one-month ordeal, he gained twenty-five pounds, and developed an array of physical ailments including nausea, depression, a splotchy complexion, nightmares, a fatty and inflamed liver, and loss of sexual desire. His cholesterol level rose 30 percent and his triglycerides doubled, and he developed high blood pressure. His overall risk of heart disease doubled in just thirty days, and he suffered from chest pains and shortness of breath. The quality of his life deteriorated along with his health. We watched this film with our children, and it was a life-changing experience for them. They have always been quite good about avoiding junk food, but this movie made them swear never to eat another French fry or drink another Coke.

Unless you have been living under a rock for the past decade, you know that a steady diet of fast food can make you fat and unhealthy. A new study from the University of Minnesota found a direct link between eating fast food and the development of type 2 diabetes. Published in the January 1, 2005, issue of *The Lancet*, this trial reported that people who consumed fast foods two or more times a week were typically ten pounds heavier than those who ate fast food less than once a week. Even more worrisome was the finding that the fast-food fans had a twofold increase in insulin resistance, which stimulates the pancreas to pump out even higher amounts of insulin and usually leads to increased belly fat and higher risks of diabetes and heart disease.

Compounding the problem is the fact that fast-food portion sizes have increased *two- to fivefold* over the past fifty years. Today, it is easy to down a whole day's calorie requirement in a few minutes and for just a few dollars. A single fast-food meal can disturb your metabolism and increase the levels of inflammation in your blood, so it is important not to binge regularly. If your vascular system is under constant siege from the effects of fast-food meals, you will be predisposed to aging and diseases like heart attack, stroke, and Alzheimer's disease.

Being mindful of how specific foods affect you is an important step in caring for yourself. We suspect that if you pay close attention, you will notice adverse effects such as fatigue, lethargy, and a drop in your ability to concentrate for a few hours after you eat foods like doughnuts, French fries, or ice cream that are high in processed carbs like sugar and white flour, and loaded with bad fats. When you are tempted by these delicious but toxic treats, think of how you will feel after you eat them rather than how great they will taste. This should be an effective deterrent to the lure of inflammatory junk foods and a reminder to opt instead for healthful natural whole foods.

3

RULES OF THE DIET

Simplicity is the essence and power of this diet. If you stick to its simple rules, most of the time you will lose excess body fat, grow younger and healthier, and improve your longevity. By following this program you can consistently make the right food decisions, and safely eat anywhere from your own kitchen to a McDonald's restaurant. The plan starts with an induction phase that generally lasts about two weeks. This strict regimen is to help wean you away from the addiction to sweets and starches. After that, you can add up to one alcoholic drink daily for women or two drinks daily for men. Ideally, it is best to limit yourself to not more than one drink a day regardless of your gender. Although you may have only one serving of whole grains per day for the first two weeks, after the induction phase most people can use up to two or three servings per day. No sugar or processed grain products are allowed. If you seem to be having a hard time losing your excess body fat, cut back to one serving of grains per day and eliminate the alcohol again.

1. Eat three or four meals daily, of approximately the same size. Use the smaller nine-inch plates rather than the standard eleven- or thirteen-inch plates.

2. You *must* eat breakfast every morning—no exceptions.

3. Consume a variety of natural fresh foods each day.

4. Eat lean protein at least three times daily, including at breakfast. The serving should be about the size of your hand. This can be more difficult than it sounds. Good protein options include fish, fowl, wild game (like elk, buffalo, and venison), fresh and lean cuts of red meat, whey protein powder, nuts, natural peanut butter, eggs, nonfat yogurt, low-fat cottage cheese, or mozzarella cheese.

5. Eat at least nine servings or handfuls of produce daily, which equals four and one-half cups per day. This should include three or four servings of fruit per day; vegetables (except potatoes) as desired, at least four or five servings daily—the fresher and more colorful the better.

6. Do not eat any white flour, white rice, potatoes, or sweets. Avoid any processed foods containing high-fructose corn syrup, hydrogenated (trans) fats, or saturated fats. For desserts, choose fruits such as berries or one to three ounces of dark chocolate. Initially, limit grain products to one serving per day of whole grain such as oatmeal—steel-cut oats or old-fashioned oats (eat raw or lightly cooked). Avoid the quick cook oats. Other options include whole-grain bread (with visible grain, seeds, nuts, etc.), air-popped popcorn, wild rice, brown rice, some breakfast cereals such as those containing no hydrogenated oils or added sugar, and at least three or four grams of fiber per serving.

7. Drink at least two cups of tea daily, preferably green tea—consider drinking some of it as decaffeinated tea. Do not have more than three cups of coffee per day; drink tea if more stimulants are needed.

8. Do not drink any alcohol (yet!). After the two-week induction phase, up to one (for women) or up to two (for men) drinks will be allowed per day. Red wine is best, but any form of alcohol will provide health benefits if consumed in moderation (not more than ten drinks per week). Avoid sugary mixes like soft drinks. If beer is your preferred alcoholic beverage, try to choose a low-carb or light beer.

9. Try to use a scoop of whey protein powder (without added carbs and mixed in water, nonfat milk, or soymilk) once or twice per day. (We prefer to use whey at breakfast and/or at the midafternoon snack.)

10. Women should try for two cups of nonfat milk daily; men should have one cup.

11. Consider adding soy to your diet in the form of unsweetened soymilk or other soy products—up to two servings daily.

12. Consume four sixteen-ounce bottles (about one liter) of water daily. You will need more if you are exercising vigorously.

13. Do not drink sugared beverages, fruit juices (low-salt vegetable juices are acceptable), or diet beverages. You will be too busy trying to drink all of the acceptable liquids to even miss the sweet drinks anyway.

14. No TV while eating. You should not have the television on during meals, and there should be no snacking while watching TV programs. No eating in front of the television, since it triggers mindless snacking in many people. Ideally, eating at home should be restricted to only one spot that isn't anywhere near the television—the kitchen or dining room table for instance.

15. Do not have any food after eight p.m. Calories that you consume within two or three hours of bedtime are less likely to be burned and more likely to end up as body fat.

16. Take the following supplements: two or three highly purified fish oil capsules per day; one multivitamin daily, containing at least 400 to 800 IU of vitamin D, as well as the daily value of most of the other essential nutrients. Women may need supplemental calcium as well. Men over age forty-five and women over fifty: Take one 81 mg aspirin daily.

Three Meals Per Day of Approximately Equal Size

According to centuries-old advice, the meal plan for staying lean and healthy is to eat breakfast like a king, lunch like a shopkeeper, and dinner like a pauper. The goal is to eat about the same number of calories for breakfast, lunch, and dinner. To be precise, the ideal proportion of calorie intake should be about 25 percent at breakfast, 30 percent at lunch, and 30 percent at the evening meal, leaving about 15 percent of calories for snacks, which are best consumed in the mid-afternoon. For most people, this means substantially bulking up breakfast and trimming down the evening meal and snacks.

Breakfast: The Most Important Meal

You will notice marked improvements in mood and energy, with fewer cravings for junk food, when you eat a breakfast that is high in water, protein, good carbs (loaded with antioxidants), and healthy fats. But many people who struggle with their weight often skip breakfast altogether or have a light breakfast consisting of something like a glass of juice with a bagel, a piece of toast, or a bowl of cornflakes. The typical American breakfast is essentially pure carbohydrate that is quickly absorbed and leads to a spike in blood sugar followed by a compensatory spike in insulin. This stimulates a steep fall in blood sugar, leaving you famished and sluggish by mid-morning and susceptible to cravings for doughnuts, pastries, cookies, and junk foods and sugary drinks from the vending machines that are ubiquitous in the workplace. This eating style is a vicious cycle that forces you to mindlessly consume excess calories leading to obesity, aging, and disease. Instead, have a Forever Young breakfast with protein (eggs, whey protein, fish, or meat) and high-nutrient, fiber-rich foods (fruits, nuts, berries, or veggies), and wash it down with tea, water, soymilk, or nonfat milk. The rest of the morning you will walk right by the box of doughnuts at work without feeling compelled to indulge yourself.

A recent paper from Vermont's Rutland Regional Medical Center confirmed decades of data showing the importance of eating breakfast each morning. This study found that the breakfast bunch received four important benefits:

1) lower BMI (average body weight)
2) reduced risks of diabetes, metabolic problems, and obesity
3) better long-term weight loss maintenance
4) improved mental alertness throughout the day

A study from the February 2005 issue of the *American Journal of Clinical Nutrition* found that people who skip breakfast tend to have a higher calorie intake throughout the remainder of the day, with worse cholesterol and insulin levels than those who eat a healthy breakfast. Breakfast jump-starts your system when you roll out of bed in the morning by increasing your metabolic rate about 25 percent. This revs your energy up and improves your ability to perform both physically and mentally. On the other hand, people who skip breakfast are stuck in the hibernation mode and are often plagued with the consequences of a slow metabolism like obesity, constant fatigue or sluggishness, and chronically feeling cold. Snacks eaten before bedtime are more likely to be converted to body fat while you sleep. In contrast, breakfast calories can be burned throughout the day supplying you with the energy you need to perform your best.

Remember, if you don't consume adequate protein for breakfast you will not be able to perform your best or resist the temptation to eat junk food throughout the morning. We often cook enough lean protein at the evening meal so that the next morning we have leftover fish, chicken, or red meat for our breakfast protein. Another option is to keep hard-boiled eggs in the refrigerator for a quick and easy protein food. Whey protein powder is another one of our favorite breakfast protein options. Natural slow-burning carbs like berries, fruits, vegetables, or a serving of whole grains will give you an energy boost that lasts throughout the morning because they are slowly digested. The fruits and vegetables that are an essential part of a great breakfast are also your best source of the antiaging, disease-fighting antioxidants and other plant-based nutrients.

As you sleep you continually lose water through your breath and your metabolism, leaving you relatively dehydrated by morning. So start rehydrating when you wake up—water and tea are ideal beverage choices for health, appearance, and performance. We also recommend that each morning you take an omega-3 supplement to feed your brain, protect your heart, and prevent inflammation. Nuts, another tasty source of good fats, are also on the menu almost every morning at the O'Keefes'—like water, you can even consume nuts during your daily commute into work.

Many people prefer starchy or sugary foods for breakfast. Personally, we have always noticed that when we eat a breakfast of processed carbs like pancakes, cornflakes, sweet rolls, or hash browns we don't feel our best an hour or two later. Joan always emphasizes the point that starch is like dessert—you have to eat the healthy things before you can even think about starch. We recommend only one to three servings of grain products daily, and these should be whole grains like oatmeal or a piece of whole-grain bread—many people prefer to include one at breakfast.

Breakfast doesn't have to take more than five to ten minutes, but it will change your outlook for the entire day. Fruit, nuts, and some low-fat dairy provide a quick, easy option that requires no preparation time but serves as a nutritious meal with staying power. One of our favorite breakfasts is berries (strawberries, blueberries, blackberries, or raspberries), cinnamon, and fresh almonds or pecans mixed in with nonfat plain yogurt. Another easy yet complete breakfast is a scoop of whey protein mixed into glass of nonfat milk or soymilk along with fresh produce (an apple, orange, or plum for example), a handful of nuts, and a cup of tea.

> **Important!** *Immediately after breakfast, keep hydrating and drink throughout the day. When Joan is out on errands and feels like she needs something to perk her up, she often drives through McDonald's and picks up an unsweetened iced tea. There are bottled unsweetened iced teas, which are also a great drink choice when you are out on the go. When James is away from home or on rounds in the hospital, he carries decaf green tea bags in his pocket and has three or four cups during the course of the day.*

Variety: The Good and the Bad

You will thrive best if you can learn to eat an array of fresh, natural foods to get the wide range of nutrients that are necessary for vibrant health. Different foods provide different nutrients, so the greater variety of nature's bounty in which you partake, the better health you will enjoy. Eat an abundance of fruits and vegetables and try new ones every chance you get. Look for brightly or deeply colored varieties as they are high in antiaging antioxidants. Look for an opportunity to participate in a Community Supported Agriculture (CSA) co-op. Typically you pay an up-front or monthly fee to have a variety of fresh seasonal produce or meat delivered from a local farm to your home each week.

Variety is also important when choosing animal protein sources. Red meat, poultry, nonfat dairy, whey protein, seafood, and fish all have very different nutritional profiles. Try not to eat the same type of meat or fish day in and day out. A mixture of protein sources will supply you with an array of healthful nutrients and still help you to avoid the overconsumption of potentially toxic substances that may be present in specific meats or fish. For instance, tuna is fine once or twice a week, but if you ate it every day, you might end up accumulating toxic amounts of mercury. Lean red meat is great in moderation, but when eaten in excess you might absorb too much iron, saturated fat, and heterocyclic amines (carcinogens). Lean chicken breasts are low in fat but don't have the beneficial omega-3 fats found in fish and seafood, or the high zinc levels of red meats.

Variety, however, has a dark side. The dramatic rise in American body weight over the past twenty-five years is paralleled by a line documenting the number of new man-made foods introduced into the diet over the same time period. They are often advertised as low fat, low carb, or vitamin-fortified, but nearly all of these synthetic, caloric-dense delicious new foods are designed to entice us into overeating. We must learn from our mistakes over the past two decades, when all fats were inappropriately identified as dietary villains. A whole host of designer "fat-free" highly processed foods were gobbled up by the American public as it packed on pounds of fat tissue faster than grain-fed cattle in feed lots. The synthetic low-carb food craze today is just the second verse of the same old song. Though the easily digestible carbohydrates are removed from these low-carb foods, they are high in calories, saturated fat, and chemicals that are completely foreign to the natural human diet.

The answer to this dilemma is to eliminate nearly all of these processed, unnatural foods from your diet since this sort of variety is detrimental. It is much easier to stay healthy by just considering this whole genre of highly processed foods off limits. Stop eating out of plastic packages and cardboard boxes, especially those with long ingredient lists that include scores of chemicals. Many of Joan's friends and clients pull their sunglasses down over their eyes and sneak into another aisle when they see her in the grocery store. She always tells her clients, "If you find yourself at the checkout with a basket full of packages and boxes, park the cart and start over!" At the supermarket stay on the perimeter and "shop the U," choosing produce, poultry, lean red meat, fish, nuts, nonfat or low-fat dairy, and whole grains. If you don't bring the junk food home, you will have a much easier time making the right choice when you eat there.

A Day Without Protein Is a Day of Aging

Adequate protein intake is a key to staying lean and young. The essential amino acids from protein provide the building blocks necessary to make or repair muscle, bone, hair, nails, and all other tissues. When your diet is insufficient in high quality biologic protein, you are susceptible to disease and aging. That's why we preach: *"A day without protein is a day of aging!"*

Studies comparing various types of diets in overweight individuals show that health benefits accrue when you lose weight regardless of how you lose it (as long as you're not taking dangerous supplements containing stimulants or picking up a tobacco addiction).

Bill Gavin, MD, is an enlightened cardiologist who authored a great little book called *No White at Night* that offers simple advice for losing weight and keeping your heart healthy: "If you eat lean protein with your meal, you will not be hungry for an additional two to three hours. I have found that it is very easy to not eat if you are not hungry. The converse is also true; it is very difficult to continue to avoid food when you are hungry, and the food choices people make for snacking are often poor. I believe that a major problem of high-carbohydrate, low-protein diets is that they make people excessively hungry between meals. Adequate protein and minimal processed carbs are crucial if you want to be able to stick with a healthy diet in the long term."

A high protein intake will ensure that exercise you do will burn off body fat rather than muscle. In the August 2005 *Journal of Nutrition* a study reported that obese women who exercised regularly lost more fat and less muscle on a protein-rich diet than those who exercised to a similar degree and ate the same number of calories but consumed a higher proportion of processed carbs. The high-protein, high-exercise group lost an average of twenty-two pounds, almost 100 percent of which came from body fat (especially around the midsection). In contrast, the high-carb, high-exercise group lost fifteen pounds, but 25 to 30 percent of this was from muscle. A protein-rich diet when combined with exercise provides synergistic benefits to improve both your body shape and composition.

The branched chain amino acids (leucine, isoleucine, and valine) are particularly critical to the metabolic advantage of a protein-rich diet. These amino acids work with insulin to build muscle. These benefits are magnified by a low–processed carb diet, which will keep your insulin levels low, allowing you to burn fat instead of sugar or muscle for energy. The richest source for these high-quality amino acids are lean protein sources like whey protein and lean animal meat.

Growing evidence shows that lean meat is not only OK, it can be among the most nutritious of foods. Lean animal protein eaten at regular intervals keeps you filled up, increases your metabolic rate (thereby burning more calories), reduces the risk of diabetes, and facilitates weight loss. Even red meat is fine if you choose lean cuts like eye of the round roast, top round steak, top sirloin steak, boneless shoulder, pot roast, round tip roast, pork tenderloin, shoulder steak, and most game meats. Trim off all visible fat before cooking. Compared to skinless chicken breast, lean red meat has only one more gram of saturated fat per three-ounce serving. But the red meat has six times more zinc, three times more iron, and eight times more vitamin B_{12}. Try to avoid highly processed and salted meats and don't cook meats at high temperatures because that produces charring and high levels of carcinogens. We suggest that you always place aluminum foil under the meat or fish that is to be grilled. By keeping the flesh food away from direct heat, you can minimize the formation of carcinogenic substances during cooking.

Overcooked meat also contains advanced glycated end products (AGEs)—found predominantly in the browned portions of meats cooked at high temperatures—that can accelerate the aging process. This is one more reason to cook at lower temperatures, using techniques such as boiling, microwaving, steaming, poaching, braising, and baking instead of frying, grilling over a direct flame, or broiling at high temperatures. Lean, fresh meat cooked appropriately is a healthy, beneficial component of a hunter-gatherer diet, especially when the meat is consumed with plenty of fresh fruits and vegetables.

Steaming Is Best

Steaming is the healthiest option for cooking vegetables and meats/fish. A study from the University of Illinois found that steaming broccoli for about three to four minutes increases the amount of sulphoraphane (a powerful cancer-fighting antioxidant) that is able to be absorbed by the body. Steaming gently and quickly tenderizes vegetables and meats/fish yet leaves their flavors and nutrients intact. It adds no calories and no carcinogens and is an ideal method for cooking most vegetables and many meats.

A Good Egg

Humans have eaten eggs for as long as we have been on the planet. They are a natural food that provides high-quality protein and a host of other vital nutrients that can help keep you strong, lean, and vigorous. Long vilified as a cause of high cholesterol and heart disease, eggs have been vindicated and today play a legitimate role in a healthy diet. Although they are very high in cholesterol, eggs are low in saturated fat, a more important determinant of your cholesterol level. Even the American Heart Association now says an egg a day is OK for anyone without cholesterol problems. And egg whites or no-cholesterol egg substitutes are a great protein source for anyone.

Joan virtually always has Egg•Land's Best "premium eggs" in her cart as she scoots around the periphery of the grocery store picking up other fresh foods. These eggs come from chickens whose diet is supplemented with flaxseed and have 25 percent less saturated fat, 15 percent less cholesterol, 22 percent more lutein, ten times more vitamin E, and three times more omega-3 fat—all for only about a dollar more per dozen. If you eat eggs, you should switch from your regular brand of eggs to one of the omega-3 enriched varieties. The omega-3 fat in these eggs is DHA—the fat that is critical for building healthy cell membranes in the heart and brain. If you have high cholesterol, we suggest that you eat only one yolk per serving of eggs to minimize the cholesterol load.

People with heart disease, diabetes, or high cholesterol should be careful about how many yolks they consume. Mark, forty-three, is a patient who required two stents to reopen diseased coronary arteries. His cholesterol had risen thirty points at the time of a recent checkup despite an excellent diet and exercise program and a statin cholesterol medication. A few months prior to that visit, Mark had read that eggs were now considered to be healthy food, and he had gotten into the habit of eating a five-egg (with five yolks) omelet each morning. Joan explained that he could use all the egg whites or egg substitute (like Egg Beaters) he wanted, but he needed to limit the intake of yolks to not more than five per week. After following this advice, his cholesterol was back under control by the next visit three months later.

Eat Fresh

As previously mentioned, you should try to consume most of your calories in the form of fresh whole foods in their natural forms, like fruits, vegetables, nuts, berries, fish, and poultry. These natural foods generally have a high nutrient-to-calorie ratio, and the higher proportion of them in your diet, the better. Eat fresh fruits and vegetables with every meal and aim for nine servings daily. A serving of vegetables is about the size of a tennis ball, and a serving size of fruit is about one-half cup. Try to consume a rainbow of colors: red (tomatoes, peppers, and watermelon), yellow (squash, grapefruit, and cauliflower), orange (carrots and oranges), green (spinach, broccoli, and green onions), and purple (beets and red cabbage). Most white foods, like white bread and white rice, are nutritionally barren and loaded with calories. However, foods like onions, garlic, cauliflower, mushrooms, and popcorn (air-popped or popped in canola oil) are among the healthiest choices of any color. Think about shopping for fruit and vegetables at several different stores to increase the variety of fresh natural foods that you bring home.

With all the confusion out there about diet, the one variable most experts can agree upon is the need to increase our intake of fresh fruits and vegetables. Only 16 percent of Americans are eating five servings of fruits and vegetables per day—almost no one is meeting the new target of nine per day.

Diets rich in brightly colored fresh fruits and vegetables are very high in antioxidant vitamins, minerals, and phytonutrients. When you get your antioxidants by consuming healthy natural foods and beverages, you will receive remarkable anti-aging and disease-preventing benefits that don't seem to occur when you try to take these nutrients in pill form. These natural foods have been linked to improved longevity, low obesity rates, reduced risks of cancer, heart disease and stroke, a healthy gastrointestinal tract, healthy teeth and bones, and reduced chance of Alzheimer's disease and other forms of dementia. When you cut carbs by excluding certain of these antiaging foods, you are throwing out the baby with the bathwater. Indeed, you must eliminate the bad carbs in sugary and starchy foods, but it is equally important to add the good carbs by consuming at least nine servings of the vegetables and fruits daily. In doing this, you will be stoking your system with anti-aging phytonutrients while at the same time, you consume fewer calories.

You will not stay young and energetic if you do not eat fruits and vegetables—lots of them. Buy fresh, eat fresh is our mantra when it comes to nutrition. Each meal should have about three servings of vegetables or fruit, preferably fresh or frozen. Many of our patients and clients tell us, "I just don't prefer to eat fruits and vegetables." We suggest they find some plants besides potatoes (the most popular "vegetable" in America) to eat regularly or get used to the idea of chronic disease and reduced longevity. Potatoes don't really count as vegetables; they are mostly starch and really belong in the bread category.

Many of the superstars of age-defying nutrition are found in the produce aisle and the frozen food section of your grocery store year-round. We are just in awe of the nutritional power of greens, and the whole family eats them on a daily basis. It doesn't get much easier or more nutritious than *spinach*; just take it out of the bag, pour on a little olive oil, and squeeze a fresh lemon over it. Then add a few other vegetables like tomatoes, carrots, cauliflower, or avocados and you have half the meal ready.

An apple a day plus a high vegetable diet are the key players in the dietary prevention of cancer. Cyanidins are antioxidants that are found in abundance in apples, red wine, and cocoa, and they appear to help to prevent cancer of the colon. The phytonutrients in the apple peel are especially beneficial, and Red Delicious and Granny Smith apples are the highest in antioxidants.

A Mayo Clinic study identified 450 men and women diagnosed with non-Hodgkin's lymphoma and compared their diets with a group of similar people without this lethal form of cancer. Three or more servings of vegetables a day—potatoes not included—reduced the risk of non-Hodgkin's lymphoma by 40 percent according to this study. The diet of the cancer-free people included about one cup daily of greens like spinach and one-half cup daily of cruciferous vegetables such as broccoli, cabbage, cauliflower, or brussels sprouts. Whole fruits, red, orange, and yellow vegetables, and processed tomato foodstuffs like tomato sauce and juice also showed protection against cancer. Don't wait to develop cancer to change your eating behavior—do it today, while you are still healthy.

> *Joan makes a habit of placing cut-up fresh vegetables and a dip like salsa out as a snack in the late afternoon. This is a great ploy to get the family to gobble up healthy produce. She also recommends this strategy in promoting weight loss. If you look, you can usually find precut and prewashed vegetables at your local grocery store.*

The second most commonly eaten vegetable in America today is iceberg lettuce, a relatively weak substitute for real antiaging vegetables like spinach and broccoli. If you eat iceberg lettuce frequently, try substituting fresh spinach or some other more nutritious leaves like romaine, kale, bok choy, collard greens, arugula, cilantro, or mixed greens. Iceberg lettuce is calorie-free and natural, and thus not a bad food.

But if you are going to eat salad, you can really stoke your system with antiaging nutrients by choosing spinach in particular. Just compare the color and consistency of iceberg lettuce and spinach and you can get a strong hint about the nutritional differences between the two. Spinach is high in beta-carotene and other antioxidant carotenoids, and it is also a good source of folate, vitamin C, fiber, calcium, and iron.

Freshness is very important to ensure that the nutrients in these foods are still intact. Natural whole foods do not contain preservatives and other artificial ingredients like trans fats to keep them fresh-tasting for months, so the nutritional content and the flavor of natural fresh foods deteriorate quickly when they become stale.

Eat Big to Get a Smaller Waist

Big foods are those that are low in caloric density, but they give you a feeling of satiety on fewer calories. Examples include salads, noncreamy soups, vegetables, fresh fruit, water, nonfat plain yogurt, fish and seafood, and cooked oatmeal. Because these natural high-volume, or "big," foods are high in fiber and water they fill you up on fewer calories than the calorie-dense highly processed foods. You are hard-wired to eat until your stomach is stretched, which generally takes about fifteen to twenty minutes. If you are eating cheese fries, chicken nuggets, and M&M's and drinking sugared sodas, during that fifteen- to twenty-minute meal, you will consume thousands of calories, mostly in the form of unhealthy and nutritionally barren foods that will be stored as belly fat and leave you hungry again in two or three hours. On the other hand, if you sit down to a meal of boiled shrimp, crisp celery sticks with guacamole dip, an apple, and a tall glass of iced tea, fifteen to twenty minutes later you will be just as full even though you consumed a fraction of the calories and loads more antiaging antioxidants, fiber, and vitamins. As a bonus, you remain full for four to six hours without cravings for junk food.

Many very healthy foods are essentially calorie-free, including spinach, broccoli, cauliflower, lettuce, and asparagus. But not everybody enjoys all the vegetables. My son Jimmy, for example, complains, "Brussels sprouts were not meant to be food. They don't taste, look, or smell like food. Whoever came up with the idea that these little shrubs were meant to be eaten by humans was mistaken." Nonetheless, all these vegetables are high in nutrients and low in calories.

Drinking calorie-free beverages such as water, tea, and coffee is another way to fill up without stressing your system with excess calories.

A High Nutrient to Calorie Ratio: The Formula to Good Health

Joan likes to teach her clients to ask themselves this simple question when trying to decide whether a particular food is something they should or shouldn't eat: "Could I find this food or drink in nature?" Water—sure, soda pop—sorry, apple—great, corn chips—no way, shrimp—perfect, chicken nuggets—wrong. Most Americans today are overfed yet undernourished, which eventually leads to obesity and poor health. The answer to this pervasive problem is simply to eliminate the low nutrient-to-calorie ratio foods like processed grains, sugars, fatty processed meats, soft drinks, and packaged snack foods, and increase the intake of high nutrient-to-calorie ratio foods like vegetables, fruits, seafood, and whey protein. A diet with a high nutrient-to-calorie ratio supplies you with large quantities of beneficial vitamins, minerals, and other antiaging phytonutrients, but at the same time it reduces your calorie intake.

If you want to be lean, fit, vigorous, and bright and happy, you must do what you are designed to do. People usually eat until they are full or satiated. If you consume natural high-nutrient but low-calorie foods like fruits and vegetables, you can eat more volume and thus will feel satisfied for a longer period after eating. It is very difficult to get fat by eating vegetables and fruit. If you also make sure to include healthy lean protein with each meal, you will stay full longer and be able to avoid cravings. It could not be simpler: Eat meals that have lots of vegetables and fruit high in fiber and water and are high in lean protein and nuts; avoid processed starchy and sugary foods, fried foods, and foods high in saturated or trans fats. Add some daily cardio exercise and include strength training (like weight lifting) and/or flexibility exercise two or three times per week and you will flourish like never before.

If you are trying to lose weight and not feel deprived, subtle changes can lead to real, lasting results. A study by Penn State researchers tested whether they could fool people into thinking they were eating the same amount of calories even though they trimmed their intake by 800 calories a day. They did this by "super-sizing" the portions of foods with high nutrient-to-calorie ratios like vegetables and fruits. At the same time they cut high-calorie synthetic foods containing sugars and fats by about 25 percent. As it turned out, the participants did not even notice that they were consuming fewer calories because they were eating more food and staying full longer. On the other hand, when the researchers cut calories by just decreasing portion sizes, participants complained they weren't getting enough to eat. In other words, you will feel less deprived and have better luck losing body fat if you increase your intake of fruits and vegetables and cut out processed high-sugar and high-fat foods, rather than relying on cutting portion size alone.

Some people do best to deprive themselves entirely of foods they crave, like sugar, bread, bagels, and pasta. These foods can be addictive—like a cigarette to a smoker or a drink to an alcoholic. Once you reintroduce them back in your system, hormones are released that make it almost impossible to resist continued use. When you eat easily digestible carbs like starch and sugar, serotonin and other "feel-good" hormones give you immediate gratification.

Nature's Energy Foods

Despite the marketing claims, energy bars and drinks are not ideal food for most athletes or other people with active lifestyles. Many contain high fructose corn syrup, other sugars, and saturated fats. When athletes ask about energy bars and drinks, we steer them instead to water, tea, nuts, berries, and dried fruits like raisins and prunes (dried plums). Oranges, bananas, apples, nectarines, grapefruits, kiwis, and whole grains are other examples of great choices for carbs before or after strenuous exercise. Nuts have healthy omega-3 and monounsaturated fats and other nutrients, so they make great energy and brain foods as well.

Shake the Salt Habit

The health of your arteries is critically important to virtually every aspect of your health. Too much salt (sodium) ages your cardiovascular system by raising your blood pressure and hardening, stiffening, and thickening your arteries and the walls of your heart. You want to keep your blood vessels soft, smooth, and supple like they were when you were a child and a teenager and avoid developing the rigid, inflamed, and crusty pipes that can lead to heart attack, stroke, and congestive heart failure.

As an American adult, your chances of developing high blood pressure during your lifetime are 90 percent. If you continue to follow your current lifestyle, sooner or later you will probably get hypertension—the medical term for high blood pressure. Why? For starters, the average American consumes about 4000 mg of sodium daily, which is about *six to ten times* more salt than we were designed to eat. Add the fact that blood pressure rises in response to too much body fat, stress, and sugar and too little sleep and exercise, and you have the recipe for high blood pressure. In February 2005, the Center for Science in the Public Interest estimated that too much sodium kills 150,000 Americans each year. Excess sodium does much more than just raise your blood pressure. A study by David Calhoun, MD, reported in February 2005 *Cardiology News* showed that high-sodium intake reduced blood vessel wall function. In addition, salt leaches the calcium from your bones, making you prone to osteoporosis and fractures, and also appears to increase cancer risk—especially in the GI tract. A recent study found that extra salt in the diet increased the likelihood of heartburn (also known as esophageal reflux) by as much as 70 percent.

A good place to start lowering the sodium in your diet is by removing the salt shaker from the table and hiding it in an inconvenient spot. But only about 5 percent of the salt in our diet comes from the salt shaker; 75 percent comes from processed and restaurant foods. Most people do not choose to eat high-sodium products—they just eat the foods that are readily available in our culture. Salt is everywhere in our modern diet, even in foods such as bread that don't taste salty. Processed foods are loaded with salt to help preserve freshness, and the more sodium you eat, the more you will crave salt. When you eliminate highly processed, high-sodium foods from your diet, you will take a huge step toward a healthier, more vigorous life.

Fresh fruits and vegetables contain virtually no sodium and thus are great for lowering your blood pressure along with your weight—we recommend at least nine servings of fresh produce daily. Unprocessed meat, poultry, and fish contain only small amounts of sodium, but the more highly processed versions like deli meats, smoked or barbequed meats, beef jerky, and other commercially modified meats are usually very high in salt. The processed snack foods are generally also high in sodium. Try to get used to eating nuts that are unsalted or only lightly salted.

Look for the sodium content on food labels and avoid items that have more than 400 mg per serving. Limit your daily intake to not more than 2300 mg (about one teaspoon)—the average American eats almost two times this much. One glass of regular V8 vegetable juice has over 1000 mg by itself (low-sodium V8 or tomato juice is great), and a single dill pickle has 440 mg. A high potassium-to-sodium ratio is one of the most important parameters of a healthy diet. We are designed to take in much more potassium than sodium, but the ratio is reversed and sodium dwarfs the potassium consumption. So how do you get more potassium? You guessed it—lots of fruits, vegetables, lean protein, and other Forever Young natural whole foods.

A Rainbow of Salt Varieties to Avoid
White salt: table salt
Red salt: ketchup
Yellow salt: mustard
Black salt: soy sauce
Green salt: pickles and olives

Tea Time

Green tea is a uniquely powerful beverage for improving health, burning body fat, and preventing disease. Today, this ancient beverage has a bright future owing to a steady stream of new studies showing the health benefits accrued by drinking it. We routinely have a cup of decaf green tea in the evening after the kids are in bed and we can relax and enjoy spending some quiet time together. We try to drink two to four cups throughout the day and find decaffeinated green tea keeps us focused yet relaxed. It is also one of the best sources of beneficial phytonutrients that are helpful in preventing aging and disease. Tea is a great way to stay well hydrated without consuming excess empty calories. Green tea increases your metabolism and appears to selectively mobilize the fat stores from inside your abdominal cavity. Regular tea drinkers have a lower risk of diabetes, high blood pressure, and heart disease.

The active components of green tea are potent antioxidants: polyphenols (or catechins) and flavonols. These compounds give tea not just its color and flavor, but also its antioxidant disease-fighting properties. The specific polyphenol that appears to be the most protective is epigallocatechin gallate (EGCG), an antioxidant that is twenty-five to one hundred times more potent than vitamins E or C. A single cup of green tea provides more antioxidant protection than a serving of strawberries, carrots, or even broccoli. In theory, this should make green tea a great tool for preventing illness like cancer, heart disease, and Alzheimer's dementia.

Green tea is one of the best sources of flavon-3-ol polyphenols. Other sources of this age-defying antioxidant include berries, apples, pomegranates, red wine, and grapes. Flavon-3-ols provide powerful multiple health benefits including protecting the LDL cholesterol from oxidation (helping to prevent plaques in the arteries); reducing inflammation; lowering the risk of cancer by inhibiting the genetic and cellular injury; and blocking aging of the skin induced by sunlight. Since we started drinking three to four cups of green tea daily, we seem to be less susceptible to sunburn.

The biologically active phytonutrients in green tea also stimulate various aspects of the immune system. Studies show that green tea does protect against DNA damage, the initial insult that can create a malignant cell. It also seems to help extinguish cancerous colonies of cells before they get a foothold in the body. Tea consumption has been linked with lower risks of cancers of the lung, colon, breast, liver, prostate, bladder, pancreas, and skin. A Mayo Clinic study published in the journal *Blood* in August 2004 found that a component of green tea suppresses the proliferation of viruses that are believed to predispose to adult leukemia. The scientific findings linking green tea to cancer prevention are so compelling that the Chemoprevention Branch of the National Cancer Institute has launched a program for the development of tea compounds as potential human cancer prevention agents.

> ### Give Your Brain a Tea Break
>
> *A steaming cup of black or green tea, the comforting drink of choice for millions of people around the world, may also help to treat or prevent Alzheimer's disease. Laboratory tests found that regular consumption of green and/or black tea inhibits the activity of certain enzymes in the brain that are implicated in the development of Alzheimer's disease. Researchers from the Medicinal Plant Research Centre at Newcastle University tested coffee as well as green and black tea, for beneficial effects in patients with dementia. This study found that coffee had no significant effect, but both black and green tea especially inhibited the activity of enzymes associated with the development of Alzheimer's. Although tea alone almost certainly will not cure Alzheimer's disease, it could possibly be another tool used to treat or prevent this increasingly common and devastating disease.*

Green tea is an excellent choice for a beverage either at mealtime, during breaks at work, or in the evening, especially if you choose decaffeinated tea. Tea contains about 50 mg of caffeine per cup compared to 100 mg per cup of home-brewed coffee and up to 200 mg per cup of espresso brewed in a specialty coffeehouse. Naturally decaffeinated tea has only a minimal amount of caffeine (4 mg). Tea contains unique highly beneficial compounds including theanine, which induces a relaxed yet focused state of mind. Unlike most antianxiety agents, theanine increases alertness and energy, yet reduces tension, worry, and negative thinking. If you could use *more* energy and focus in your life with *less* anxiety and mental stress, incorporate a few cups of green tea into your daily routine.

Green Tea for "Good Abs"

Belly fat is not just unbecoming, it is very dangerous to your long-term health and well-being. When excessive fat is stored inside your abdominal cavity it has devastating metabolic consequences. This intra-abdominal adipose tissue continually dumps fatty acids into the bloodstream poisoning your muscles so they become unresponsive to the normal action of insulin. That means your insulin, sugar, cholesterol, and blood pressure levels go up, predisposing you to high blood pressure, diabetes, heart disease, and even some forms of cancer. Finding a way to selectively burn this toxic belly fat has been the holy grail of scientists and dieters alike, but it has proved to be an elusive goal.

Evolving evidence points to green tea and its components like theanine and cat-echins as at least part of the answer to this problem. A study documenting the effectiveness of tea for burning body fat in men was published in the January 5, 2005, issue of the *American Journal of Clinical Nutrition*, and a recent animal study found that the equivalent of four cups of green tea daily improved exercise endurance by increasing the body's ability to burn fats for energy.

You will need to drink about three to four cups of either caffeinated or decaf-feinated green tea per day to see the full benefits including weight loss, increased metabolism, and a shrinking waistline. Following the other aspects of the Forever Young diet and exercise plan will improve the fat-burning and age-reversal benefits of this wonderful drink.

Tea and Fluoride

The tea plant naturally concentrates fluoride from the soil and water. Instant tea is a reasonably good choice of beverage, although in very large quantities (more than two or three quarts daily), it can result in excessive fluoride intake. Brewed tea also contains fluoride, though in lower concentrations than instant tea. Additionally, brewed tea is higher in antioxidant phytonutrients than instant tea and thus is prefer-able when available. The fluoride in tea is not necessarily a bad thing. Tea consump-tion has been linked with healthier teeth and gums and stronger bones, possibly in part due to its fluoride content. Fluoride is not a concern unless you are drinking more than two or three quarts of instant tea, or a gallon of regular brewed tea, daily.

Coffee or Tea?

Coffee is America's favorite stimulant. There are over 167 million regular coffee drinkers in the United States, which translates into about 60 percent of the adult population. According to Joe Vinson, PhD, at the University of Scranton in Penn-sylvania, Americans get more of their beneficial antioxidants from coffee than any other dietary source. The one and two-thirds cups of coffee the typical American consumes each day provides about 1300 mg of antioxidants. The next richest source for antioxidants was tea at 294 mg per day. Although cup for cup tea is higher in antioxidants, Americans drink much more coffee each day. This study, presented in August 2005, reported that between coffee, tea, wine, and beer, Americans drink about 60 percent of the total antioxidants they consume each day.

Coffee is quite habit forming due to its pleasant aroma and flavors, as well as its high caffeine content. Daily coffee consumption leads relatively quickly to a mild—and for most people, a usually harmless—form of chemical dependency. Symptoms of caffeine withdrawal—headache and lethargy—appear predictably within only twenty-four hours of caffeine abstinence. Yet many people do not tolerate even moderate doses (above 50 or 100 mg) of caffeine without experiencing adverse side effects. The formal definition for "caffeine intoxication" is a dose of 240 mg, which is typically obtained in just two cups of brewed coffee. If you can use coffee without suffering undue side effects like anxiety, jangled nerves, insomnia, jitteriness, and palpitations, you can safely drink two to three cups a day guilt free.

Recent population-based studies suggest that coffee may help prevent diabetes and liver cancer and may reduce risks for degenerative brain disorders such as Parkinson's disease and Alzheimer's disease. Two large studies (involving over 200,000 patients total) published in the July 6, 2005, issue of the *Journal of the American Medical Association* looked at the role of coffee in preventing diabetes. The researchers concluded that two to four cups of coffee daily reduced the risk of developing diabetes by about 30 percent. Of note, even decaffeinated coffee appeared to help prevent diabetes. Low-fat or non-fat milk is a healthy additive for you coffee. On the other hand, adding cream and or sugar to your coffee will erase some of the benefits.

Despite the growing evidence of the health benefits of coffee, based on scientific evidence and our own personal experience, we feel strongly that green tea is a much healthier choice than coffee for a daily stimulant. Even decaf green tea provides substantial stimulant effects owing to its content of theanine and other stimulants in addition to small amounts of caffeine.

Many people find the energy jolt and mood-lifting effects of caffeine indispensable in their day-to-day existence. Moderation is the key to navigating the fine line between enjoying the mood and productivity boost from a mild "caffeine buzz" and avoiding the negatives like insomnia, the jitters, and irregular heartbeats. Tea has about one-third or one-half the caffeine of coffee, and thus is a more moderate choice for your stimulant. Many of our patients and clients drink a cup or two of coffee in the morning, change over to green tea for the afternoon, and then decaf green tea in the evening. Avoid adding sugar, artificial sweeteners, and nondairy creamers (loaded with trans fat) to your tea and coffee.

Here's to Your Health:
The Case for and Against Alcohol

Alcohol is a classic double-edged sword in relation to human health. Scientific studies consistently suggest that low to moderate intake is beneficial to your health. Increasingly impressive data indicate that your health will be substantially better if you drink a little alcohol every day than if you don't drink at all. Observational studies indicate that drinking small to moderate amounts of alcohol can decrease the average person's risk of dying during any given year by as much as 25 percent. A review of the major studies on the effects of alcohol was published in the *Southern Medical Journal* in the summer of 2004. The authors concluded that one alcoholic drink daily was the dose that conferred the maximum health benefits. At that intake, the heart protection is highest and the risks for alcohol-related health problems are at their lowest. People who drink one or two drinks daily have a 25 to 50 percent lower risk of heart attack, a 40 percent lower risk of stroke, and about a 33 percent reduction in the risk of developing diabetes.

However, heavy alcohol use devastates not just your health but often your personal and professional life as well. Research shows that the risks of oral and esophageal cancer, cirrhosis and cancer of the liver, colon and breast cancer, atrial fibrillation, and fatal motor vehicle accidents all go up in proportion to alcohol intake above about two drinks per day. Alcohol is also high in calories that—like those in sugar—tend to end up around your abdomen. Heavy alcohol use is often associated with nutritional deficiencies as well.

Exactly what constitutes a "drink"? James once saw a retired maître d' who admitted (only at the prompting of his wife, who was seated next to him in the exam room) that he drank a bottle of red wine nightly. James urged him to cut his intake to not more than two glasses per night. Three months later, he proudly announced that he had, in fact, cut back to two glasses nightly. James noticed his wife rolling her eyes and asked her what kind of glasses he was using. She replied in an irritated tone, "Twelve-ounce tumblers. He's still downing a bottle nightly, except now it takes him only two glasses to do it!" So for the record, a drink is defined as five ounces of wine, twelve ounces of beer, or one and a half ounces of distilled spirits like whiskey, vodka, gin, or rum.

A glass of red wine is probably the best way to get the benefits of drinking because of its potent antioxidant flavonoids and polyphenols that come from the purple grape pigments. These antiaging compounds in red wine and deeply pigmented plants help to quell the fires of inflammation. A study published in the July 2004 issue of the journal *Atherosclerosis* compared red wine and gin for reducing inflammation. Results showed that the red wine drinkers had lower levels of C-reactive protein (CRP), an important marker of inflammation and a risk factor for heart attack. A study in the January 9, 2003, issue of the *New England Journal of Medicine* found that men who drank alcohol at least three or four days of the week had a significantly decreased risk of heart attack. The benefits seemed to be related to frequent but modest consumption of alcohol and are mostly attributable to the ethanol, which raises the protective HDL cholesterol, makes the blood less likely to clot abnormally, and appears to even decrease the risk of developing diabetes when used in moderation. Dry red or white wines are lower in sugar and calories and thus are healthier choices than sweeter wines. Similarly, light or low-carb beers and unsweetened mixed drinks are better for you than the sweeter versions of these beverages.

Much of the health benefit of moderate drinking may be related to its stress-relieving antianxiety effects. Happy and healthy usually go hand in hand. Sitting down at happy hour to unwind and emotionally connect with important people in your life can help to make you more relaxed and improve your overall health. Studies do show that alcohol seems to be most protective when it is consumed daily, in moderation, and before or during the evening meal. Still, we do not recommend non-drinkers take up alcohol unless they can be sure it will not turn into a problem. You should abstain from alcohol completely if you have a personal history or a strong family history of chemical (alcohol or drug) dependency or severe liver disease.

The Sharp, Double-Edged Sword

Some people rationalize their occasional overindulgence by saying, "All things in moderation; even moderation!" For the record, moderate drinking is anywhere from 1 to 10 drinks per week for women and 1 to 14 drinks per week for men. No, you can't save them up all week to justify a ten-drink binge on Saturday night.

Let's be perfectly clear—getting drunk on the weekends is not heart healthy or good for any other aspect of your health. Binge drinking or chronic excessive alcohol use wreaks havoc with your well-being. A new study by Robin Room, PhD, showed that alcohol abuse kills as many people around the world as tobacco and high blood pressure. This study in the February 5, 2005, issue of *The Lancet* states that alcohol causes about 4 percent of worldwide deaths, playing a role in more than sixty different medical conditions. By comparison, tobacco is responsible for 4.1 percent and high blood pressure, 4.4 percent of deaths. Data from the World Health Organization show that alcohol abuse is responsible for about 1.8 million deaths worldwide each year. In the United States alone, 75,000 people die yearly from excessive alcohol intake.

Since the early 1990s, binge drinking (usually defined as five or more drinks during one session for a man and four for a woman) has increased by almost 30 percent and is especially common in young people on and around college campuses. Portion control with alcohol consumption, like eating food, is critical to good health. Women who have more than one drink daily have an increased risk of breast cancer. However, a high intake of folic acid (folate) appears to make this alcohol-related breast cancer risk disapper entirely. So if you drink alcohol regularly, make sure you also take a daily multivitamin and eat a diet high in folate-rich foods like spinach, broccoli, and asparagus.

Daily alcohol consumption is a slippery slope that many people cannot safely navigate. As someone with a strong family history of alcoholism, James knows from personal experience that from a societal perspective, alcohol use probably causes more suffering than health benefits. Nowhere in health is the double-edged sword as sharp on both sides as it is with alcohol. A little each day can make you healthier and happier, but too much can ruin and/or shorten your life. If you can limit your consumption to not more than one or two drinks per day, alcohol can be something that adds both life to your years and years to your life.

BENEFITS OF MODERATE ALCOHOL INTAKE

Disease	Effects of Drinking Alcohol
Heart Attack	Men who drink five to seven days weekly have a 37 percent lower risk.
Diabetes	Risk of developing new diabetes is 34 percent lower in regular drinkers. People with established diabetes have been shown to have a 60 percent decreased risk of heart attack if they drink regularly, compared to people with diabetes who don't drink.
Stroke	One to two drinks per day has been associated with a 40 to 60 percent lower risk of stroke. Higher intake increases stroke risk.
Dementia	One to three drinks per day has been associated with a 42 percent lower risk of dementia (including Alzheimer's disease).
Osteoporosis	Women who consume six or seven drinks weekly have a higher bone density than nondrinkers. However, women who drink more have increased risk of osteoporosis.

Source: *Southern Medical Journal*, July 2004

Tip: *Using a tall thin glass when drinking alcoholic beverages is a reliable way to decrease portion size. People predictably overestimate how much fluid is in a tall slender glass compared to short wide glass.*

The Water of Life

Water has the power to rejuvenate you just like the rains revitalize the desert. It naturally keeps beautiful things beautiful. Your body is 70 percent water, your brain is 85 percent, and your blood is 90 percent water by weight. Vibrant, shiny, dewy, hydrated, and moisturized: Water is what makes you and every other living thing on Earth feel and look alive. It is not just an excellent way to improve skin appearance, but it is also essential for healthy kidney, heart, blood, and brain function.

When oral cravings occur, drink pure water either from a reputable bottled source or a good under-the-sink or household water filter. This should be the default beverage that you consume throughout the day. Carry bottled water in the car at all times. Think of bottles of water like your keys—you aren't going anywhere without them. We keep a case of bottled water in the trunk of our car. Take advantage of the time behind the wheel by doing something good for your body, like meeting your hydration needs.

A study of the Seventh-Day Adventists showed that those who drank five or more glasses of water daily had half the heart disease deaths and fatal strokes than those who drank less water. If you really love carbonated drinks such as sugared sodas or artificially sweetened drinks, you should try sparkling water with a refreshing slice of fresh lemon or lime. Potent antioxidants called limonenes are present only in the peel of citrus fruit, making sparkling water with a refreshing slice of lemon or lime.

You have probably read and heard much about the quantity of water that is recommended but less about its quality. Chlorine is a potent biotoxin that is added to water in a dose large enough to kill germs but not people—at least not in the short term. However, it makes sense that once the chlorine has done its job and killed the microbes, we should get this potentially dangerous compound out of our water before we drink it. We have a filter that removes essentially all of the chlorine and other contaminants from our household water before we drink or bath in it. If you rely on bottled water, make sure to use a high-quality brand that has been purified with reverse osmosis and has been tested and found to be free of impurities. Some brands are nothing more than tap water in a bottle. Even with a filter for your drinking water at home, it is a good idea to keep some bottled water on hand to use when you are away from home, exercising, or driving around in the car.

Drinking generous amounts of water on a day-to-day basis helps you lose weight. Scientists do not entirely understand why a high water intake causes weight loss, but it clearly does. You will burn off ten pounds of flab over the next year if you do nothing else but drink sixty-four ounces of water daily. Admittedly, it's a myth that you need to consume the proverbial eight cups of water a day to stay healthy. More recent guidelines emphasize *total* water intake, which includes beverages other than pure water and the water found in foods. These recommendations still conclude that we need about sixty-four ounces of water daily, but you can get it from many other sources besides plain water—for instance, a small tossed salad contains about six ounces of water. Indeed, the average American gets about 70 percent of his or her hydration from food and beverages other than water, and that's OK if you are not overweight and not working out vigorously. But if you are carrying around extra weight that you would like to shed or you just want to look and feel better, water is your friend.

A German research team measured the resting metabolism of healthy men and women before and after they drank sixteen ounces of water. Their metabolism began to rise within just ten minutes of drinking the water, and by forty minutes, their average calorie-burning rate was 30 percent higher, and it stayed higher for an hour. Cool or cold water works best for weight loss, because the calorie-burning effect comes from having to heat the water up to 97.8 degrees like the rest of the water in your body. In fact, the formal definition of a calorie is the amount of energy required to raise the temperature of a liter of water by one degree Celsius.

Water is a deceptively powerful antiaging beverage: It rehydrates your tissues making you look, feel, and act younger. Pure water also contains no calories or free radicals; therefore, when you drink sixty-four ounces or more a day, it displaces many other unhealthy items like soda in your diet. Replace just two cans of regular soda with two refreshing glasses of plain H_2O and eliminate 300 calories. If you can make this a daily routine, by the end of one year you will be up to thirty pounds lighter.

Water is the ultimate sports drink, too. Unless you are exercising vigorously for more than sixty to ninety minutes, water is the best fluid to use for staying hydrated and improving performance and overall health. Most sports drinks are loaded with chemicals like salt, sugar, artificial colors, preservatives, and caffeine. While it is true that you lose sodium when you sweat, this is a good thing. We tend to consume six times more sodium than we really need, predisposing us to high blood pressure, stroke, and osteoporosis. Drinking high-sodium, high-calorie beverages like Gatorade negates some of the benefits of a good hard workout, because you *want* to burn off some excess calories and flush out excess sodium and toxins. Drink plenty of pure water before, during, and after exercise, especially if you are sweating profusely. Think of it like changing the oil in your car: out with the bad, in with the good.

If you want to lose weight, you will have to drink more than one quart of water daily. Body fat is a very lightweight, efficient mechanism for storing energy, but you need to add water, a lot of it, to unlock those calories. A single pound of body fat contains about 3,500 calories, enough to keep you alive (in starvation mode) for four days. But to burn that pound of fat, you will need to drink about nine pounds of water above your baseline requirements.

In summary, the goal is eight glasses (eight ounces each) of water daily. Bottled, clean spring, filtered, or sparkling water (with a twist of citrus or a splash of juice) are ideal.

High Fructose Corn Syrup—a Key Ingredient in the Recipe for Obesity

Caloric soft drinks—pop, Coke, or soda—are sweetened with high fructose corn syrup (HFCS). The stuff is ubiquitous in our modern food supply, and it is one of the compounds that may be poisoning your system, making you insulin resistant and overweight, and predisposing you to diabetes, heart disease, and possibly even cancer. In the *American Journal of Clinical Nutrition* in April 2004, an article analyzed food intake patterns by using U.S. Department of Agriculture food consumption tables from 1967 to 2000. The intake of HFCS had increased more than 1,000 percent between 1970 and 1990, far outstripping the changes in intake of any other food or food group. This chemical now represents more than 40 percent of caloric sweeteners added to foods and beverages. Americans are consuming about 200 to 300 more calories per day than they were three decades ago, and between one-half to one-third of these are in the form of HFCS. In 1966, we consumed no HFCS; today the average American consumes sixty-three pounds of the toxic stuff per year!

In the Midwest, we see trains pulling black tanker cars filled with tons of HFCS being shipped to food manufacturers around the continent. They love high fructose corn syrup because it is cheap, protects foods from freezer burn, keeps products fresh-tasting, and improves their shelf life—but it will shorten *your* shelf life. HFCS is six times sweeter than old-fashioned white table sugar. All of the various soft drinks that contain sugar rely on HFCS as the "natural sweetener." Candy bars, commercial baked goods, most breads, and most sweetened junk foods (like those that fill vending machines and line the aisles of convenience stores) also contain HFCS.

How HFCS Fuels the Obesity and Diabetes Epidemics

It is no coincidence that the increased use of HFCS in the United States mirrors the rapid increase in obesity. The digestion, absorption, and metabolism of fructose differ from those of other sugars like glucose and sucrose. HFCS is not taken up and burned by the muscles but instead is shunted to the liver. There it is immediately made into triglycerides causing a spike in these dangerous fats that are damaging to the arterial walls when they peak quickly, as they do after a meal or drink high in HFCS. Researchers discovered long ago that the surest and quickest way to make a laboratory animal insulin resistant is to feed them HFCS. Within days to weeks of consuming a diet rich in HFCS, these high triglyceride levels poison the muscles by making them insulin resistant.

Almost one of every two adults has insulin resistance, which is probably the most important health problem facing Americans today. It causes most high blood pressure, almost all diabetes, much of the heart disease and stroke, and even many forms of cancer. As ominous as all these diseases sound, most people can rationalize them away with the "it won't happen to me" mind-set. But what really motivates them is the knowledge that insulin resistance is destroying their youthful glow and sexy figures. It ruins the complexion by predisposing to acne and a puffy, bloated, pitted skin appearance. People with insulin resistance often have a paunch and weak, atrophied arms and legs. If you want to recapture the look and vigor of your youth, defeat insulin resistance and you will thrive and glow again.

In addition, unlike glucose, fructose does not stimulate leptin production. Since leptin is a hormone that signals the brain that you are full, dietary fructose, particularly in beverages, may encourage caloric overconsumption and contribute to increased weight gain. In other words, drinking soda will not decrease your hunger the way other foods and drinks do. As Greg Critser points out in his excellent book *Fatland*, the overuse of fructose is skewing the national metabolism toward fat storage and away from calorie burning.

HFCS now makes up about 10 percent of the average American's daily calorie consumption and up to 20 percent of the typical child's diet. This accounts in part for the growing epidemic of type 2 diabetes in children and teens. The biggest source of HFCS for most Americans, especially young people, is soda pop. In the second half of the 1980s, the large soft drink franchises like Coca-Cola and Pepsi-Cola aggressively moved into the country's high schools. This brilliant marketing strategy utilized incentive contracts whereby a school would get upward of $100,000 annually from the soft-drink company for the exclusive right to sell and market their beverages on campus. From 1989 to 1994 when this marketing force was unleashed on the schools, the average teen consumption of soda increased 70 percent. Today the average teenager in America drinks about sixteen ounces of soda per day, or over fifty gallons per year. Studies show that for every twelve ounces of soft drink per day your child drinks, his or her chances of becoming obese increase about 60 percent! If you drink one soda a day for a year, it adds up to 58,400 extra calories—or about seventeen pounds. Therefore, one of the first and most important things you and your family should do is to quit consuming soda and other foods and drinks sweetened with HFCS.

Quit Drinking All Sodas!

If you can get a handle on what you are drinking, you will be well on the way back to your ideal weight. In a trial from Purdue University, researchers found that calories consumed in sweet liquid form predisposed subjects to overeating more than solid food. Participants were given an extra 450 calories either in the form of soft drinks or jelly beans. The people who ate the jelly beans later consumed almost exactly 450 fewer calories than before, whereas the soda group ate about the same amount of calories they normally did and consequently gained weight. The researchers speculated that the liquid calories in the soda do not seem to register with your body's automatic calorie counter that helps us to regulate our appetite.

If you prefer a fizzy beverage, unsweetened sparkling water is a great option because it does not contain phosphorus or the other artificial ingredients found in soft drinks. If you depend on Coke and other caffeinated sodas to keep you energized, tea is a perfect alternative. If you make this trade, you lose the empty calories, appetite stimulators, and phosphorus (that leaches calcium from your bones). Instead, you are taking in a calorie-free drink that increases your metabolism and is rich in antiaging disease-fighting antioxidants.

The Bitter Truth About Artificial Sweeteners

Ronnie is a bright, successful forty-five-year-old man who has struggled with his weight his entire life. Because he has blockages in his coronary arteries, James has been working with him for the past few years to get his risk factors in line. At five seven, 275 pounds, he was more than 100 pounds overweight. James had a long talk with him about the right diet and lifestyle, and he seemed committed to making real changes. A year later at his annual visit, they were both frustrated to see his weight up to 290 pounds. James was amazed to learn that Ronnie has been drinking about *two liters* of *diet colas* daily. Although aspartame, the noncaloric sweetener that he consumes in large quantities, is calorie free, it indirectly contributes to his inability to lose weight.

Joan has noticed that many of her clients who seem to have the hardest time keeping their weight under control are the same people who drink the most sugar-free soft drinks. Surprisingly, scientists have never been able to show that using sugar substitutes helps people to lose weight. In fact, the latest studies indicate just the opposite: Artificial sweeteners make you prone to overindulge in other sweets, the calorie-loaded kind, by interfering with your body's natural ability to gauge calories based on the sweetness of a food or drink. So while these sugar substitutes offer the weight-conscious person a calorie-free sweet treat, they also sabotage their weight-loss efforts and fuel an addiction to sweets.

The artificial sweetener industry is doing a booming business in America the "Waist-land." When you walk down the aisles in the supermarket, you are barraged with brightly colored banners touting "diet" this, "no-sugar-added" that, and "low-carb" other things. While the overconsumption of sugar and other processed carbs is probably the most serious problem with the American diet, these sugar substitutes are not a great option either. The rise in the use of artificial sweeteners is directly linked to America's dramatic rise in obesity. The population that regularly uses artificially sweetened sugar-free products has grown from 70 million in 1987 to over 160 million in 2000. During that same time period, the number of overweight Americans doubled. *Paradoxically, it is as if the more calorie-free Diet Coke or Diet Pepsi you drink, the more weight you gain.* Before the recent appearance of sugar substitutes, a food's sweetness provided reliable clues about its caloric content—the sweeter it was, the more energy it contained. In the modern era, we are losing the ability to judge a food or drink's calorie content based on the sweetness. In one study published in July 2004 in the *International Journal of Obesity*, researchers confirmed this, reporting that the use of a sugar substitute had impaired rats' natural ability to compensate for the calories in a sweet snack.

There are many factors contributing to the unprecedented weight gain in America over the past thirty years, and the use of artificial sweeteners is just one piece of the puzzle. Undoubtedly, part of the reason that the increase in weight tracks with the use of artificial sweeteners is that overweight people are more likely to try to cut calories. Still, sugar substitutes will not help you lose weight and may even worsen the problem.

These sugar substitutes seem to encourage the addiction to sweet foods and drinks that vexes many overweight individuals. Legitimate questions do exist about the safety of some of them (stevia, saccharin, acesulfame), and you would definitely be better off without them. But whatever you do, don't use this as an excuse to go back to drinking regular sodas sweetened with HFCS. These are even worse because they contain calories *and* stimulate your appetite for yet more sweets. If you really need a carbonated beverage, switch over to sparkling water with a slice of fresh lemon or lime, or flavored but unsweetened sparkling water. This is what we do around our house, and even the kids don't miss the sweet sodas at all.

The New American Guidelines on Diet and Exercise

In January 2005, the federal government released its new dietary and exercise guidelines accessible on the Internet at www.healthierus.gov/guidelines/. These are updated and revised every five years as a cooperative venture between the Department of Health and Human Services and the Department of Agriculture. This latest version is a marked improvement over the previous somewhat misguided recommendations which, for example, suggested that Americans try to eat eleven or more servings of grain products per day—a formula for obesity. The new guidelines are remarkably enlightened, hit fairly close to the mark, and deliver a pretty clear message. The brightest and best minds in the field are finally coming to a consensus about the ideal program. The focus is on more fresh vegetables and fruit, moderate amounts of legumes, whole grains, and lean protein, smaller serving sizes, and avoidance of high-calorie sweet, starchy, and fatty processed foods, as well as getting about thirty to ninety minutes of moderate or vigorous physical activity daily. The bad news is that the average American is light-years away from meeting these recommendations. Two out of three of us are overweight, less than 5 percent consume nine servings of produce daily, and only one of three meets the minimum goal of thirty minutes of exercise daily. Still, it is important to know what the ideal goals are so we can set our sights on the right objectives.

We feel that the suggested intake of low-fat or nonfat dairy at three servings daily is too much. The recommendation of six servings of grain products daily is also too high in our estimation. And the protein intake is somewhat less than we suggest. Still, most other recommendations are very reasonable, and if you follow them, you will probably lose weight and improve your long-term health.

The New Food Pyramid

1. Exercise at least thirty minutes daily (or most days) to reduce the risks of heart disease, diabetes, osteoporosis, and other common diseases of aging. The activity can be done in shorter segments, as long as it adds up to at least thirty minutes per day. Adults should aim for about sixty minutes of moderate to vigorous physical activity most days to prevent weight gain. Those trying to lose weight or maintain weight loss may need up to ninety minutes of exercise per day.

2. Consume at least nine servings of produce daily (five or more servings of vegetables and four servings of fruit per day). A serving of vegetables is one cup of raw green leafy vegetables like spinach, or one-half cup of cut raw or cooked vegetables.

3. Daily protein intake should be about six ounces.

4. Eat or drink three cups of dairy each day.

5. Fats should be limited to 20 to 35 percent of calories. Focus on healthy fats like omega-3 and monounsaturated fats.

6. Sodium intake should be less than 2300 mg daily, or about one teaspoon of salt daily.

7. Alcohol intake of up to one drink daily for women, and two drinks daily for men, is recommended. (One drink equals five ounces of wine, twelve ounces of beer, or one and a half ounces of distilled spirits.)

8. Eat about three (and not more than six) servings of whole grains daily.

How Does One Get Nine Servings of Vegetables and Fruit in a Day?!

For most produce, a half cup or a handful is one serving; double the serving size to one cup, and you get credit for two servings of vegetables or fruit. In other words, you need to eat about four and one-half cups of produce per day. For example, eat half of a grapefruit and a bowl of oatmeal with either a half cup of berries or half a banana for breakfast, and that's two servings out of the way before you leave home in the morning. At lunch, eat a salad of one cup of greens and one-half cup of vegetables with an apple for dessert. Have a pear for a midafternoon snack, and for dinner include one cup of steamed vegetables. You've hit the magic number of nine servings of produce for the day. Our family (kids included) manages to make it most days.

You could also try to have a piece of fruit or a serving of vegetables every two or three hours during the day. This will keep your stomach filled up and your body stoked with disease-fighting, antiaging phytonutrients that are abundant in plant foods. Studies show that if you snack exclusively on produce rather than soft drinks, chips, and candy, you can expect to lose about one pound of body fat per week.

4

EATING THE
FOREVER YOUNG WAY

Unlike most diet books you won't find a large section on recipes in this book—for the most part, we don't use them. Simple and natural are the fundamental characteristics of the Forever Young diet. Recently, we camped out in our basement for eight months while our thirty-year-old kitchen was being updated. We found that we missed our oven and stove surprisingly little, despite the fact that we continued to eat at home about six evenings each week. Grilled fish, meat, or poultry with two to four servings of fresh vegetables and fruit makes a delicious and extremely healthy meal that is easy to prepare. In general, the more complicated the preparation process, the less healthy the food. For example, Joan doesn't bake at home because baking starts with white flour, sugar, and butter. With ingredients like those, the end result is a recipe for weight gain, aging, and heart disease. And to make matters worse, the smell of chocolate chip cookies in the oven is virtually irresistible. So while you miss out on the homemade cookies, you end up enjoying life more. As Joan likes to tell her clients: "Nothing tastes as good as thin feels."

Complicated dishes usually contain a host of unhealthy components like high-fat cheese, butter, cream, and salt, so you can save yourself time, get rid of your excess body fat, and grow healthier by just keeping it simple. Of course, we make exceptions. As Thanksgiving approached this year, Jimmy worried that grilled turkey served with raw tomatoes, carrots, spinach salad, steamed broccoli, and cranberries for desert just didn't seem like enough of a Thanksgiving feast. To his relief, we were invited over to the home of close family friends, and they served mashed potatoes and dressing; but the roasted turkey, sweet potatoes, green beans, and salad also fit in nicely with our natural food diet.

Suggestions for Healthy Food Choices

In order to help you move away from your current, probably less-than-ideal diet, we've provided some meal plans and guidelines so you can get started on the Forever Young diet. With practice, this simplified eating plan will become second nature. You will look and feel better, and you will also have more time for family and the other activities in your life.

Breakfast
Protein options
> One scoop of whey protein (in water, soymilk, or nonfat milk)
>
> Eggs (two whites, one yolk) or three egg whites
>
> Peanut butter (two tablespoons)
>
> Nuts (one handful, with your fingers lightly touching the heel of your hand)
>
> Lean red meat (two to four ounces)
>
> Chicken breast, fish, or turkey (two to four ounces)
>
> Salmon (smoked or lox) (two to four ounces)
>
> Cottage cheese (one cup)
>
> Nonfat yogurt (no added sugar is preferable; one cup)
>
> String cheese (two small)

Whole grain
> Oatmeal (one-half to three-fourths of a cup)
>
> Cold cereal (at least two and preferably three or more grams of fiber per 100 calories; no hydrogenated fat)
>
> Whole-grain toast (three or more grams of dietary fiber per 100 calories)

Dairy
> Eight ounces of nonfat milk. If lactose intolerant, consider calcium-fortified soymilk for women, noncalcium soymilk for men.

Also include:
> One or two servings of fresh fruits or vegetables
>
> One to two cups of tea or coffee

Morning hydration

At least twenty-four ounces of water and one cup of tea (iced or hot)

Lunch

Lean protein source. For a quick, easy lunch cook more protein than you need the night before so that you have some leftover meat, poultry, or fish for the next day's breakfast or lunch.

Vegetables as desired—at least two

One fruit. Try to avoid too much fruit at lunch since the higher load of sugar, even in the form of fruit, can produce an early afternoon drop in alertness and energy.

Water and tea, the more the better

Afternoon snack (if you are feeling true hunger)

It is generally best to have this snack in the midafternoon from three p.m. to five p.m. Try to include a protein food like a scoop of whey protein in water, nonfat milk, or soymilk. A protein food for the midafternoon snack helps to curb the appetite at dinner and in the early evening hours, when most people are likely to overeat.

Examples of afternoon snacks

Whey protein drink with a serving of fruit or vegetables

One string cheese with a piece of fruit

Peanut butter on an apple

A handful of nuts with a piece of fruit or a vegetable

Vegetables dipped in salsa (each as much as you want)

Drink throughout the afternoon: Twenty-four ounces of water and a cup of hot or iced tea (mandatory)

Dinner

Lean protein source

Two or more servings of fresh fruit or vegetables

Women need eight ounces of nonfat milk; men should drink water, tea, or non-calcium soymilk.

When your goal weight is achieved, feel free to add a five-ounce glass of wine (preferably red) and/or a whole-grain snack at dinner.

Sample Menus
Day 1

Breakfast

One cup of plain nonfat yogurt mixed with a handful of almonds or pecans, a teaspoon of ground cinnamon, and a half-cup berries or a quarter cup of raisins

One scoop of whey protein in a cup of water, soymilk, or skim milk

One cup of tea or coffee (optional)

During the morning drink twenty-four ounces of water and one cup of tea (mandatory)

Lunch

One-half of a roast beef sandwich (about three ounces of meat, one slice of whole-grain bread)

Fresh vegetables dipped in salsa

One-half of a grapefruit

One cup of skim milk

During the afternoon drink twenty-four ounces of water and a cup of decaf green or black tea (mandatory)

Snack

One pear, 1 small cheese stick

Dinner

Boiled shrimp

One cup of edemame (steamed soybeans) in the shell

Cole slaw salad with vinaigrette

Three-fourths cup cantaloupe

Water or skim milk and/or decaf green or black tea

Decaf tea and/or water throughout the evening as desired

Day 2

Breakfast
> Scrambled eggs (one yolk, two whites per person) with chopped tomato
>
> One slice of whole-grain toast with one teaspoon of Benecol or Take Control margarine
>
> One-half of a banana
>
> One cup of skim milk
>
> One cup of tea or coffee (optional)
>
> During the morning drink twenty-four ounces of water and one cup of tea (mandatory)

Lunch
> Boiled shrimp and half of an avocado with fresh lemon juice squeezed over the shrimp
>
> Three-fourths cup strawberries
>
> One apple
>
> One cup of tea or water
>
> During the afternoon drink twenty-four ounces of water and a cup of decaf green or black tea (mandatory)

Snack
> One scoop of whey protein in a glass of water, soymilk, or skim milk

Dinner
> Split pea soup
>
> Spinach salad with vinaigrette
>
> Grapes (twelve is a standard serving)
>
> Water or skim milk and/or decaf green or black tea
>
> Decaf tea and/or water throughout the evening as desired

Day 3

Breakfast
> Old-fashioned oatmeal (slightly undercooked, not mushy), with one-half cup of pecans and one-half cup of berries or one-half of a banana
>
> One scoop of whey protein in water, skim milk, or soymilk

One cup of tea or coffee (optional)

During the morning drink twenty-four ounces of water and one cup of tea (mandatory)

Lunch

Tomato slices, mozzarella cheese, and basil drizzled with balsamic vinegar

Five dried plums

During the afternoon drink twenty-four ounces of water and a cup of decaf green or black tea (mandatory)

Snack

One orange and a handful of nuts

Dinner

Baked salmon with lemon wedges

Steamed green beans

One-half to three-fourths cup canned peaches packed in water or their own juice

Cucumber, green onion, and cauliflower salad with vinaigrette dressing

Skim milk or water or decaf green or black tea

Decaf tea and/or water throughout the evening as desired

Day 4

Breakfast

Half a grapefruit

Unsweetened high-fiber cereal with skim milk, one-half cup of berries, and one-quarter cup almonds or pecans

One scoop of whey protein in water, soymilk, or skim milk

One cup of tea or coffee (optional)

During the morning, drink twenty-four ounces of water and one cup of tea (mandatory)

Lunch

Salad of spinach, baby carrots, raw almonds, raw broccoli, or any other vegetables you prefer, dressed with extra virgin olive oil and the juice of half a fresh lemon

Leftover baked salmon or meat

One cup of skim milk or soymilk

Apple for dessert

During the afternoon drink twenty-four ounces of water and a cup of decaf green or black tea (mandatory)

Snack

Berry smoothie (blend one cup of frozen berries, one cup of skim milk, one scoop whey protein, six ounces of skim milk, one-quarter teaspoon of cinnamon)

Dinner

Brisket cooked on low heat since morning

One cup steamed snow peas

Sliced raw tomatoes

Mixed greens salad with olive oil and red wine vinegar

Skim milk or water and/or decaf green or black tea

Decaf tea and/or water throughout the evening as desired

Day 5

Breakfast

Two hard-boiled eggs

Two kiwi fruits

Half a banana

One scoop of whey protein in water, soymilk, or skim milk

One cup of coffee or tea (optional)

During the morning drink twenty-four ounces of water and one cup of tea (mandatory)

Lunch

Leftover brisket from night before

One slice of whole-grain bread with a slice of tomato, onion, and spinach on the sandwich, plus mustard or horseradish as desired

One-half to one cup of frozen or fresh berries

One cup of skim milk

Snack

Five dried plums (prunes)

One handful of nuts

During the afternoon drink twenty-four ounces of water and a cup of decaf green or black tea (mandatory)

Dinner

    One-quarter roasted chicken, skin and visible fat removed

    Steamed mixed vegetables

    Sliced watermelon

    Dessert of fresh strawberries with one ounce of dark chocolate (at least 70 percent cocoa solids)

    Skim milk or water and/or decaf green or black tea

    Decaf tea and/or water throughout the evening as desired

Day 6

Breakfast

    One scoop of whey protein in water, soymilk, or skim milk

    One slice of whole-grain bread toasted and spread with one or two tablespoons of natural peanut butter

    Grapes (twelve is a standard serving)

    One cup of tea or coffee (optional)

    During the morning drink twenty-four ounces of water and one cup of tea (mandatory)

Lunch

    Leftover chicken from night before

    Mixed greens or spinach salad with a variety of vegetables, one-quarter cup of walnuts and vinaigrette dressing

    One orange

    During the afternoon drink twenty-four ounces of water and a cup of decaf green or black tea (mandatory)

Snack

    One small handful of mixed nuts

    Ten cherries

Dinner

    Pork chop (lean)

    Tomatoes

    Steamed zucchini

One cup of skim or soymilk

Decaf tea and/or water throughout the evening as desired

Day 7

Breakfast

One slice of whole-grain toast with two to three ounces of turkey

One-half of a grapefruit

One scoop of whey protein in water, soymilk, or skim milk

One cup tea or coffee (optional)

During the morning drink twenty-four ounces of water and one cup of tea (mandatory)

Lunch

Fast-food restaurant salad with grilled (not fried) chicken and vinaigrette or other low-fat dressing

Iced tea

Apple

During the afternoon drink twenty-four ounces of water and a cup of decaf green or black tea (mandatory)

Snack

Five dried plums (prunes)

One-half cup low-fat cottage cheese

Dinner

Chinese stir-fry (with no added oil) with steamed shrimp or chicken and vegetables, no white rice (one-half cup of brown rice is acceptable)

One peach

Skim milk or water and/or decaf green or black tea

Decaf tea and/or water throughout the evening as desired

Practical Weight-Loss Tips

1. Never eat in front of a screen (TV or computer).
2. Never eat in the car.
3. Always sit at the same spot in the house (for example, the dining room or kitchen table) when you are eating anything.
4. Never eat after 7:30 p.m.
5. After dinner, brush your teeth. This is your signal that you are done eating for the day.
6. Only eat until you are 80 percent full. Remember it takes about twenty minutes for the stomach to tell the brain that it is full.
7. Eat very slowly.
8. Drink a bottle or a large glass of water before each meal.
9. Many calories come from beverages. Stick to water, tea, some coffee, and skim or soymilk.
10. Choose the smaller (nine-inch) dinner plate for your meals.
11. Stick to three meals and one snack daily.

Some of the Healthiest Foods on the Planet

Spinach	Dried plums (prunes)
Broccoli	Apples
Grapefruit	Onion and garlic
Green tea	Fish and seafood
Berries	Whey protein
Red wine	Purified fish oil
Pomegranates	Tree nuts
Tomatoes	Pure water
Kiwi fruit	Soybeans and soy foods
Beets	Extra virgin olive oil
Avocado	

Some of the Worst Foods on the Planet

1. Anything with hydrogenated fats (transfats), most commonly found in doughnuts, French fries, commercial baked goods, potato chips and other snack foods, and stick margarines
2. High fructose corn syrup (HFCS), most common sources include sweetened sodas and candy
3. Salt
4. White flour
5. Refined sugar and almost anything that contains it
6. Saturated fat (found in fatty animal products and high-fat dairy)

The Polymeal: A Formula for a Healthy Cardiovascular System

Dr. Oscar Franco and colleagues reported in the December 18, 2004, issue of the *British Medical Journal* that making a daily habit of eating fruits and vegetables, fish, garlic, dark chocolate, and almonds, and drinking a glass of wine will reduce the risk of heart disease by up to 76 percent and significantly improve life expectancy. This diet, referred to as the "Polymeal" by the authors, represents a combination of edible items that individually have been shown to protect against heart disease. The authors concluded: "Following the Polymeal promises to be an effective, nonpharmacological, safe, and tasty means to increase life expectancy and reduce heart disease across the population."

Although modest wine consumption was predicted to afford the most impressive protection, omitting any one of the components of the Polymeal resulted in a small decline in predicted benefit. The intake of five ounces of wine daily was estimated to decrease heart disease risk by nearly one-third, and fish four times weekly reduced the risk by about 14 percent. If consumed daily, this recipe for a healthy cardiovascular system was estimated to improve longevity by about six and a half years for men and five years for women. The Polymeal is precisely the style of eating that is consistent with the Forever Young plan. Also, take notice that there are *no* starchy foods in this Polymeal plan. Think of starches like bread, bagels, rice, and potatoes as desserts, and don't eat these foods until after you have eaten all the good stuff first.

Antioxidants: Valuable as Food but Less Effective as Pills

Science can be a confusing business to the average person. For example, over the past several years the importance of antioxidant vitamins in preventing heart disease and cancer has been emphasized. However, a string of recent scientifically rigorous studies have shown no benefits from the use of high-dose antioxidant supplements such as vitamin C, vitamin E, beta-carotene, and folic acid.

Oxidative stress is still an important factor in aging and disease, but our strategies to control it are evolving. Coronary risk factors including age, hypertension, diabetes, high cholesterol levels, smoking, emotional stress, and obesity are all associated with increased oxidative stress. This means these risk factors essentially cause a "rusting" of our cardiovascular system, and predispose us to heart attack, stroke, and death. It seems logical that antioxidant vitamins might be good at preventing oxidative stress and thus cardiovascular disease, but unfortunately, vitamin supplementation studies thus far have not borne this out.

In contrast, studies about dietary antioxidants continue to show convincing benefits. It now appears that the best way to protect your system against oxidative stress is to get your antioxidants in the form of foods and drinks rather than pills. An antioxidant-rich diet is good for your heart for many reasons.

The following list outlines foods that are rich in antioxidants and have been shown to improve many parameters of cardiac health. Try to incorporate as many of these foods as possible into your daily eating pattern. The antioxidant content and activity of these foods are listed in descending order, with the foods highest in antioxidant concentrations at the top of the list.

The Top-Twelve Antioxidant Foods/Drinks

1. *Berries.* Blueberries, blackberries, cranberries, raspberries, and strawberries are all high in antioxidants and rich in healthy fiber and minerals. Berries (and nuts) are nature's ideal snack foods.

2. *Beans.* Red kidney beans, pinto beans, small red beans, and black beans. Besides being rich in fiber, folate, and magnesium, beans are near the very top of the list in antioxidant concentration.

3. *Green Tea.* One study after another shows potent benefits for tea in preventing cardiovascular events, improving survival after heart attack, and improving blood vessel function.

4. *Prunes (dried plums).* California growers have changed the name to dried plums to update the prune's image. By any name, this food is an easily accessible, inexpensive antioxidant powerhouse. We recommend four or five dried plums as an occasional snack. They are naturally rather high in sugar so use them for dessert or when you feel the urge for a sweet treat.

5. *Greens.* Spinach, kale, collard greens, beet greens, wheat and barley grasses, broccoli, brussels sprouts, and other green leafy vegetables are packed with antioxidants and are virtually calorie-free. Freshness is particularly important for maintaining the nutrient content of greens.

6. *Brightly Colored Fruits and Vegetables.* The dark and brightly colored pigments in artichokes, carrots, tomatoes, red, orange, yellow, and green peppers, broccoli, apples, plums, cherries, watermelon, pomegranates, and other fruits and vegetables are potent natural antioxidants.

7. *Red Wine.* The dark pigments in red wine, like those found in berries and other fruits and vegetables, provide antioxidant activity. It appears that the benefits of alcohol (like exercise) are temporary and thus only a small amount should be consumed daily.

8. *Olive Oil.* Extra virgin olive oil is loaded with antioxidants that have been shown to be cardioprotective, so try to incorporate olive oil into your daily diet. The FDA has recently given its stamp of approval to the claim that olive oil, at about two tablespoons daily, may reduce risk of developing heart disease.

9. *Dark Chocolate.* The dark pigments in chocolate have been shown to be strong antioxidants.

10. *Onions and Garlic.* Both of these foods contain high levels of allicin, a great antioxidant. Several studies show health benefits, including reduced cardiovascular risk factors, in people who eat these foods regularly.
11. *Soy Products.* Foods and beverages (except soy sauce) made from soybeans are very high in antioxidant phytonutrients. Try to eat one or two servings of soy daily.
12. *Nuts.* Pecans, walnuts, hazelnuts, and Brazil nuts are high in antioxidants.

5

HOW EXCESS CALORIES AND "CARBAGE" CAN TRASH YOUR HEALTH

Man was not meant to live on bread alone; in fact, we were not designed to live on bread at all. The Forever Young eating style is a low-glycemic load diet, which means it essentially eliminates easily digestible, processed carbohydrates. These calorie-dense sugary and starchy foods taste good to us because we are genetically programmed to minimize the chances of dying from starvation. Even during seasons of abundance, virtually none of the foods in the natural human diet were pure sugar or starch. If you accidentally filled your diesel car with unleaded gasoline, you would not be surprised when it ran poorly. The most important reason to avoid "carbage" like sugar, white flour, and highly processed foods is that they are foreign to our genetic makeup. Trying to stay healthy and vigorous and look lean and youthful while eating the standard American fare is as futile as trying to keep a rabbit healthy on a meat-based diet. Rabbits aren't meant to eat meat, and you aren't meant to eat pure sugar and starch.

Our excessive intake of sugar and starch, coupled with the decrease in physical activity, is at the root of the epidemics of obesity and diabetes in America. The glycemic index is a ranking of carbohydrates (from 1 to 100) based on their immediate effect on blood sugar (glucose). This term has become a real buzzword among the carb-conscious dieters, but glycemic load, the glycemic index multiplied by the carbohydrate content, is more relevant. For example, some vegetables like carrots or pumpkins have a high-glycemic index, but a low-glycemic load, and thus are not a problem if you are trying to watch your weight. For everything you need to know about glycemic index and glycemic load, go to www.glycemicindex.com.

Today, low-carb, high-protein foods are selling like hotcakes used to. While some of these are acceptable in limited quantities, you are better off filling up on nature's versions of low-carb foods: low-glycemic-load vegetables and fruits, nuts, berries, lean protein, and water. Carbohydrates are fuel for an active lifestyle. They are the only energy source your brain can burn, and they are essential for sustained physical exertion. However, the type of carbohydrate consumed makes all the difference. Upward of 50 percent of the calories the average American consumes in a day are in the form of added processed sugar and high fructose corn syrup. Most excess sugar is stored in the body as fat, particularly around the midsection. This is one of the major reasons why two out of three Americans are overweight and struggling to lose their belly fat. It is nearly impossible staying lean, healthy, and happy on this very unnatural high-sugar diet.

The Problem with Processed Carbohydrates

You probably have no idea how much the remarkable power of your diet exerts on the most fundamental aspects of your life. Your mood and energy level, how well you solve problems, how hungry you are, and the foods you crave are all profoundly influenced by what you are or aren't putting into your mouth on a frequent basis. Modern eating patterns rely heavily on the high-glycemic-load foods that are quickly absorbed and raise your blood glucose level. For many people these foods are a chemical and emotional addiction. When you eat a diet high in sugar and starch, you become emotionally dependent upon this sugar rush and constantly crave sweet foods and drinks. This high-glycemic-index diet will not only make you fat, especially around the midsection, it will also disturb your normal hormonal balance and make you chronically tired.

Too much sugar, HFCS, and other processed carbs fuel the fires of insulin resistance and inflammation throughout your body, leading to obesity, heart disease, arthritis, Alzheimer's disease, dental and gum disease, and diabetes among many other "diseases of aging." The salvation from this fate is to embrace an active lifestyle and a natural diet of fresh foods like vegetables, fruits, fish, lean poultry, nuts, berries, legumes, whole grains, whey protein, water, and tea, while strictly avoiding highly processed foods.

Insulin and You

Insulin is a critically important hormone that is abnormally high in up to half of American adults. It is produced in the pancreas, which continually monitors your blood glucose. After a carbohydrate meal, your blood glucose rises, stimulating the release of insulin, which encourages muscle and liver cells to sop up this extra sugar in the bloodstream. When simple carbohydrates become the primary form of food intake, your body tissues become numb to the normal effects of insulin. These elevated insulin levels make it more likely that the carbohydrates you eat will not get into the muscles to be burned for energy but instead end up being stored in fat cells.

The key to developing a fit and trim body is to keep your insulin levels down, and the best way to accomplish that is to avoid sugar, starch, and all foods with a high glycemic index. If you then add exercise, especially in a program that has both strength and aerobic training components (like weight training and walking), you will see dramatic improvements in your waist size, muscle strength, sleep, appearance, energy, blood pressure, cholesterol, and your overall health.

An easy way to know if you have insulin resistance is to simply check your fasting glucose level and get a cholesterol profile (total cholesterol, triglycerides, HDL and LDL cholesterol levels). Insulin resistance is usually present if you have a fasting sugar above 100, triglycerides over 150, HDL cholesterol level less than 40 for men, or less than 50 for women, blood pressure above 130/80, and waist circumference of over thirty-five inches for women or over forty for men.

Natural foods such as nonstarchy vegetables and fruits provide healthy carbs to fuel your passions and pursuits, but they won't disrupt your normal glucose-insulin metabolism. As a bonus, these natural carbohydrates are the principal sources for the beneficial age-erasing phytonutrients, vitamins, minerals, and fiber. Carbohydrate intake stimulates the release of serotonin, a feel-good chemical that generates a sense of fullness and happiness. Many people become addicted to this carbohydrate rush by eating excessive amounts of sweets and starches throughout the day. You must eliminate these foods to break this addiction and get back to a fit and healthy lifestyle. However, you can get the same feelings of happiness and satiety from good carbs like vegetables and fruits with low glycemic indices.

If you need another reason to avoid sugar and processed carbs you may be shocked to know that eating too many refined carbohydrates during the three months before conception doubles your risk of delivering a baby with a birth defect. If you are obese and are consuming a large amount of sugar and starch before conception, the risk of birth defects is quadrupled.

Diabetes and Insulin Resistance

Diabetes is probably the most important health epidemic today. The prevalence of diabetes has increased by over 100 percent over the past fifteen years. Children born today have a one in three chance of developing the disease in their lifetime, and this figure is increasing every year. Type 2 diabetes (95 percent of all cases) is caused mainly by obesity, or excess fat tissue, especially in and around the abdomen. Your chances of developing this problem rise dramatically as your weight climbs. Today, even young people (including teenagers) are developing this devastating disorder.

Diabetes is usually associated with a cluster of risk factors like obesity, high blood pressure, and abnormal cholesterol levels. We keep lowering the number when it comes to the ideal glucose. Now we diagnose diabetes when the fasting blood sugar is consistently above 126. Borderline diabetes begins when the fasting glucose is above 100. You can prevent or improve diabetes with exercise, weight loss, and diet, and there are several promising medications, including metformin, rosiglitazone, and pioglitazone, that improve your body's sensitivity to insulin, rather than just bludgeoning your system with ever higher insulin doses to combat diabetes. If you have the disease, you will also likely need an ACE inhibitor and a statin (cholesterol-lowering drug).

Insulin resistance might be your worst enemy. Almost half of us suffer from this condition that most doctors don't know how to diagnose. It causes diffuse inflammation throughout the body, and is readily apparent in the skin where it predisposes to blemishes, puffiness (fluid and salt retention), and a pitted, unhealthy complexion, as well as darkly pigmented skin around the neck, groin, and underarm regions.

Research is now showing that a high-antioxidant, low-processed carbohydrate diet such as the Forever Young program is the best way to improve your complexion. More importantly, getting insulin resistance under control will help to burn your belly and back fat, lower your blood pressure, and improve your lipids. Keeping your insulin sensitivity normal helps to prevent diabetes and dementia and is a fundamental step toward ensuring a healthy and vigorous future.

Ways to Stay Diabetes Free and Healthy

1. **Exercise.** *Both weight training and aerobic exercise markedly reduce the risk of type 2 diabetes.*

2. **Relax.** *Emotional distress can raise stress hormones, including cortisol and adrenaline, that elevate blood sugar level.*

3. **Coffee and tea.** *These drinks help to increase your basal metabolic rate, which in the long run can reduce risk of type 2 diabetes by keeping your weight down, your energy up, and your sugars in the normal range.*

4. **Modest alcohol intake.** *In a Boston University study, those who had approximately twenty drinks per month were 66 percent less likely to have insulin resistance (the underlying cause of type 2 diabetes) compared with nondrinkers.*

5. **Avoid high fructose corn syrup, sugar, and processed grains.** *HFCS, sugar, and starches can worsen insulin sensitivity and increase risk of diabetes and obesity.*

6. **Choose healthy plant-based oils over animal fats.** *Adding healthy fats such as olive oil, canola oil, and fish oil to your diet will reduce the overall risk of cardiac problems, obesity, and diabetes.*

7. **Load up on colorful fresh produce.** *A Harvard study published in* Diabetes Care *found that a diet rich in yellow, orange, and green leafy vegetables seemed to reduce risk of diabetes.*

8. **Whey protein and nonfat or low-fat dairy.** *Intake of whey protein, nonfat dairy and/or low-fat dairy has been shown to reduce weight and risk of type 2 diabetes.*

9. **Cinnamon.** *Cinnamon has been shown to improve the body's response to its own insulin, thus lowering risk of diabetes. It is a perfectly natural sweetener that can substitute for sugar.*

10. **Get your sleep.** *Studies show that sleep deprivation, especially less than five or six hours of sleep per night, can increase stress hormones, raise blood sugar and insulin levels, and thereby increase the risk of type 2 diabetes.*

11. **Avoid certain medications.** *If possible, avoid certain medications including steroids (like prednisone), old-fashioned beta-blockers (such as atenolol, metoprolol, nadolol, and propranolol), and high-dose diuretics (fluid pills).*

Fat Chance

Today many people have a hard time losing weight in part due to a slowing metabolism and a disturbed hormone profile. This is why you could get away with eating the standard American diet when you were a skinny teenager but you can't today. Too many calories increase the damaging oxidation process. Too many easily digestible carbohydrates increase the insulin level, stimulate your appetite, and increase fat deposition especially in the abdominal area. Too much stress elevates cortisol, which compels you to eat constantly and also deposits fat around your belly. Sedentary living blunts growth hormone production, whereas vigorous physical exercise is the best way to increase adult growth hormone levels, which give a powerful boost to energy, vigor, and a youthful appearance. Realigning your hormone profile by following the recommendations of the Forever Young program also provides many other antiaging benefits such as an improved complexion, more lean muscle, less male pattern balding, stronger bones and teeth, improved sex drive, better sleep, fewer nighttime awakenings to empty your bladder, more energy, better memory, and a happy focused state of mind.

Americans are getting heftier and heftier. The proportion of overweight or obese children ages six to eleven doubled between 1980 and 2000 and tripled among adolescents ages twelve to seventeen. Even older Americans are becoming plump; today seven out of ten people between ages fifty-five and seventy-four are overweight, which is about twice the prevalence thirty years ago. A study of 73,000 adults published in the *American Journal of Preventive Medicine* in December 2004 showed that having excess body fat significantly increased risk for a wide range of problems, including coronary disease, heart failure, blood clots in the veins, high blood pressure, depression, sleep disorders, indigestion, erectile dysfunction, arthritis, hip and knee replacements, asthma, and diabetes. The June 14, 2005, issue of *The Lancet* published a paper that found that obesity accelerates aging by destroying telomeres—the caps on the ends of chromosomes that prevent the DNA from fraying. In this study of 1,222 British women, the telomere shortening indicated that obesity caused about 8.8 years of accelerated aging as compared to the lean women. These increased health problems and premature aging are largely due to disturbances in hormonal and chemical balances in the body and brain often seen in overweight and obese individuals. Adding insult to injury, obesity also unfairly affects job salary. Sociologist Dalton Conley, PhD, found that in women, but not men, every 10 percent increase in weight (measured by BMI) correlated with a 6 percent decrease in income. So it's very important that you get your eating and lifestyle under control and get back to a healthy weight range.

Your Ideal Body Weight

The most widely used tool for calculating ideal body weight is the Body Mass Index (BMI), which is essentially a ratio of your weight to height. The BMI is an accurate tool for assessing whether or not you weigh too much; however, it is not perfect. Many times young body builders or athletes in strength sports such as weight lifting, football, and wrestling have an elevated BMI, but a low percentage of body fat, because they are much more muscular than the average person.

The average American has a BMI of 27.2 kg/m^2 (kilograms per meters squared); well above the healthy target BMI of approximately 18 to 25. An ideal BMI for most people is in the range of 19 to 23. In his *Real Age* books Dr. Michael Roizen has calculated that if you can keep your BMI between 18 to 23, your real age is as much as eight years younger than if your BMI is at the national average of 27.

Simply measuring the waist size is also an important marker of obesity since the most dangerous and detrimental fat is that which is deposited inside your abdominal cavity. By the way, your belt size is not always an accurate indicator of your waist circumference, especially in men who typically wear their belt somewhere south of their true waist. As a rule of thumb, the waist is the part of the body

KNOW YOUR BODY MASS INDEX													
Body Mass Index (Kg/m²)													
19	20	21	22	23	24	25	26	27	28	29	30	35	40
Height						Body Weight in Pounds							
4'10"	91	96	100	105	110	115	119	124	129	134	138	143	167	191
4'11"	94	99	104	109	114	119	124	128	133	138	143	148	173	198
5'	97	102	107	112	118	123	128	133	138	143	148	153	179	204
5'1"	100	106	111	116	122	127	132	137	143	148	153	158	183	211
5'2"	104	109	115	120	126	131	136	142	147	153	158	164	191	218
5'3"	107	113	118	124	130	135	141	146	152	158	163	169	197	225
5'4"	110	116	122	128	134	140	145	151	157	163	169	174	204	232
5'5"	114	120	126	132	138	144	150	156	162	168	174	180	210	240
5'6"	118	124	130	136	142	148	153	161	167	173	179	186	216	247
5'7"	121	127	134	140	146	153	159	166	172	178	185	191	223	255
5'8"	125	131	138	144	151	158	164	171	177	184	190	197	230	262
5'9"	128	135	142	149	153	162	169	176	182	189	196	203	236	270
5'10"	132	139	146	153	160	167	174	181	188	195	202	207	243	278
5'11"	136	143	150	157	165	172	179	186	193	200	208	215	250	286
6'	140	147	154	162	169	177	184	191	199	206	213	221	258	294
6'1"	144	151	159	166	174	182	189	197	204	212	219	227	265	302
6'2"	148	155	163	171	179	186	194	202	210	218	225	233	272	311
6'3"	152	160	168	176	184	192	200	208	216	224	232	240	279	319
6'4"	156	164	172	180	189	197	205	213	221	230	238	246	287	328

that is the first to enter a room as you walk through the doorway. To measure your waist size, place a tape measure around your body at the level of your belly button. A waist circumference of over thirty-five inches for a woman or over forty inches for a man is a serious health warning sign because excessive fat around the midsection is usually associated with inflammation of the blood vessels and increased risk of cardiovascular disease, diabetes, and high blood pressure.

To determine your waist to hip ratio, measure your waist as outlined above, and then measure your hips at their widest point, generally done by wrapping the tape measure around the area where you can feel your hip bones. Then divide your waist circumference by your hip circumference. This should be less than 0.85 for a woman and less than 0.95 for a man.

Your body mass index (BMI) is the ratio of weight to height expressed in units of kilograms per meter squared. To estimate your BMI, find your height in the left-hand column. Move across the row to your weight. The number at the top of the column is the BMI for your height and weight.

If you want to be more precise about your exact BMI, follow these instructions:

1. Convert your weight in pounds to your weight in kilograms by dividing your weight in pounds by 2.2.
2. Convert your height in inches to your height in meters by multiplying your height in inches—not feet—by 0.0254. (For example, if you are 5 feet tall, your height is 60 inches, or 1.52 meters. If you are 6 feet tall, your height is 72 inches, or 1.83 meters.)
3. Square your height in meters (that is, multiply your height in meters by itself).
4. Divide your weight in kilograms (the number you obtained in item 1) by the number you obtained in item 3. The result is your BMI.

A Lean Horse for the Long Run

James was chatting with his patient Sammy about his weight. He emphasized that Sammy's heart problems, diabetes, arthritis, cholesterol, and sleep apnea would all be markedly improved if he could shed some of the 100 pounds of excess body fat he was carrying around. Sammy snapped back, "All you doctors these days are too skinny. Look at you; you wouldn't last one minute in a bar fight." James just laughed and responded, "Sammy, how many 300-pound eighty-year-olds do you know?" In our line of work, we are constantly reminded about the importance of staying lean and fit by countless studies appearing in our journals each month and also by watching how obesity worsens the long-term health of our patients, so we are pretty good about practicing what we preach. In fact, we recently conducted a survey of about 800 U.S. cardiologists and found that only 8 percent were obese compared to about 30 percent of the American adult population.

Fans of horse racing understand that the lean horse generally wins the long run. Excess weight handicaps your chances of staying healthy and hinders your longevity. When you lose weight on a diet and exercise program like the Forever Young plan, most of the important health parameters improve in proportion to the weight lost.

Fat tissue is not just a passive storage site for excess calories; it is a highly active endocrine organ that pumps out vast amounts of important hormones and other crucial chemicals. Just like adrenal glands make epinephrine and ovaries generate estrogen, fat tissue secretes at least 25 or 30 hormones and other chemicals that regulate a wide array of critically important functions like appetite, blood pressure, mood, and growth of fat and other tissues. As metabolically active as these glistening yellow and brown globules packed inside your belly are, you might think that they would burn a lot of calories. Well, they don't. Fat cells consume just a fraction of the calories that more active cells like muscle or brain cells burn.

Adiponectin is an unusual hormone from fat tissue in that it is beneficial and positively influences your chances of staying young and healthy. Naturally, fat cells make more adiponectin when they are small and not bloated with fat. You want to keep your adiponectin level high by staying lean and physically active because this hormone fights off insulin resistance, high blood pressure, and diabetes.

A recently discovered hormone named resistin does just the opposite; it rises in proportion to your body fat. Resistin impairs your body's response to insulin, causing elevations in insulin levels and blood sugar and may eventually lead to high blood pressure and diabetes. Fat cells also churn out a number of dangerous cytokines, which are chemical messengers that are associated with inflammation that can cause heart disease, cancer, asthma, diabetes, and most of the diseases of modern civilization. Maybe the strongest factor in determining your level of inflammation and risk of developing diabetes is simply how much excess abdominal and truncal fat you are carrying around. Obesity is one of the most common causes of elevation of C-reactive protein (CRP)—a marker of inflammation that also signals an increased risk for heart disease and diabetes.

Excess fat tissue increases the levels of stress hormones like adrenaline (epinephrine and norepinephrine), angiotensin, aldosterone, and cortisol. Chronic elevation of these dangerous chemicals can increase blood pressure and the risks of heart attack and stroke, Alzheimer's, dementia, and diabetes.

Fewer Calories—More Life

For decades, scientists have known that the single most powerful and reliable technique that enables animals in captivity to live longer, healthier lives is to simply restrict their caloric intake. Studies consistently show that by reducing calorie intake by 20 percent, life expectancy can improve by 20 to 50 percent in experimental animals—from mice to chimpanzees. These studies have yet to be replicated in humans and won't be any time soon because of the time it would take to complete such a trial. However, hypocaloric diets (wherein you consume fewer calories than you burn on a daily basis) will not just reduce weight, they will also improve blood pressure, cholesterol, triglycerides, glucose, and inflammation levels and reduce risks of diabetes, heart disease, stroke, dementia, arthritis, and most other diseases of aging.

Animals and humans living in the wild ate a calorie-restricted diet by design. Natural food sources in their raw state tend to be lower in calories than our processed foods, and wild creatures work hard for every calorie they consume. Excess calories tend to "gum-up" your metabolic machinery. Your body uses oxygen to burn food the way your car's engine uses oxygen to burn gasoline. During these chemical reactions, the energy generated is harnessed and used to power your body or your car. In both cases, the combustion of fuel creates waste by-products that can cause problems if they accumulate. Your body, as a function of normal metabolism, constantly churns out toxins that can promote aging and disease. When you consume a natural diet loaded with beneficial phytonutrients and antioxidants and burn all the calories you eat, your body is able to effectively neutralize or eliminate these by-products. In contrast, chronic overfeeding with high-calorie, low-quality foods like sugar, white flour, and HFCS markedly increases the amount of oxidant stress and disrupts your normal hormonal balance. The excess accumulation of toxic by-products causes oxidation or "rusting" in your organs and tissues, resulting in chronic generalized inflammation and accelerated aging. Very overweight or obese people are literally "stewing in their own juices." Many people end up on more and more drugs and supplements to try to counteract these aging and disease-producing effects, but a much more logical and effective strategy is to simply reduce your excessive calorie intake.

The fast-food and soft drink megacorporations spend billions of dollars on marketing propaganda to brainwash us into believing that their high-calorie junk food and sugary drinks somehow make our lives happier and more exciting. The truth is exactly the opposite: A calorie-restricted diet is one of the best ways to restore your health and vigor and improve your longevity. By eliminating excess calories while eating high-nutrient fare, you may improve your life expectancy and also be able to live your entire life with zest and youthfulness.

The Science of Calorie Restriction

Calorie-restriction science dates back to 1935, when Cornell scientist Clive McCay made the surprising discovery that rats fed a calorie-restricted diet lived nearly 30 percent longer than those on an ad-lib diet wherein they could eat as much as they desired whenever they wanted.

Researchers speculate that a close relationship exists between calorie consumption, the rate of the aging process, and gene patterns. A calorie-restricted diet may improve health and longevity by a number of mechanisms: It reduces free radical production, thereby increasing resistance to stress, and it improves immunity and reduces inflammation. These issues may be important in protecting against a number of illnesses such as cardiovascular disease and cancer that cause debility and early death. If the animal evidence can be extrapolated to humans—and that is still a big "if"—calorie restriction may add from eight to ten years to the life span. The animal studies suggest that for every excess calorie you forgo, you may increase your life span by about thirty seconds. The followers of calorie restriction like to point out that for every slice of pizza you eat above what need, you give up three hours of life. If you skip that extra slice, you might just get those three hours back. A nutrient-rich but calorie-restricted diet like the Forever Young program can dramatically lower risk factors for many of the diseases of aging. A calorie-restricted diet has been shown to reduce cholesterol levels and improve blood glucose levels in animals, and now it appears the same is true for humans.

RISK FACTORS IN 18 PEOPLE ON A CALORIE-RESTRICTED DIET VS. 18 SIMILAR PEOPLE ON A TYPICAL AMERICAN DIET

Risk Factor	Calorie-Restricted Diet	Typical American Diet
BMI (weight divided by height)	20	26
Total Cholesterol	158	205
LDL Cholesterol	86	127
HDL Cholesterol	63	48
Triglycerides	48	147
Systolic Blood Pressure	99	129
Diastolic Blood Pressure	61	79
Fasting Glucose	81	95
Fasting Insulin	1.4	5.1
CRP (Inflammation)	0.3	1.6
Carotid Artery Thickening	0.5	0.8

Source: Adapted from theheart.org, April 21, 2004

Beyond Longevity: How to Eat a Low-Cal High-Nutrient Diet

Cutting calories is not a strategy that is likely to get you to your 120th birthday, but it may help you stay more youthful longer. However, the public has been rapidly moving in the exact opposite direction. Obesity is now challenging smoking as the number one cause of disease and premature death in our society. Our penchant for calorie-dense foods like sugar and processed junk foods and fast foods is one of the main reasons that two out of three adults are now overweight or obese. Eating predominantly highly nutritious low-calorie food is the logical way to practice calorie restriction. A few "life extensionists" follow a calorie-restricted diet solely to live longer. Many more Americans, however, are trying to do so simply to lose weight, but perhaps the best reason to eat this way is to stay healthy and youthful longer.

Eating a Calorie-Restricted Diet

According to the Calorie Restriction Society, the underlying premise of calorie restriction is, "to eat fewer calories, while not consuming fewer vitamins, minerals, and other components of a healthy diet, and by doing so achieve a longer and healthier life." The Centers for Disease Control reports that the average adult man consumes about 2,745 calories daily, and the average woman 1,833 calories. The members of the Calorie Restriction Society aim to gradually reduce that number by about one-third.

The way to accomplish that involves lots of fruits and vegetables, and lean sources of protein like lean red meat, fish, poultry, eggs, and whey. Whole grains such as oats, barley, and legumes are also valuable sources of nutrients and fiber. They should be eaten in moderation, however, due to their relatively high calorie content. The ideal way to start cutting calories is to substitute healthy fruits and vegetables for refined carbs. Next, substitute lean protein for the fatty versions. And you won't find soda or other sweet high-calorie drinks or even fruit juices flowing from the fountain of youth. Pure clean water is nature's perfect beverage to help you stay youthful. Exercise is also essential in the equation to hold back the aging process. It is a good idea to have your cholesterol and blood glucose levels as well as your blood pressure checked at baseline so you can track your progress on a calorie-restricted diet.

Some people have tried to achieve calorie restriction through fasting. Studies do show that fasting will improve various metabolic parameters like blood pressure, lipids, and sugar. However, most people have a difficult time doing it successfully. For example, James becomes irritated even when he has to skip breakfast once or twice a year to have blood tests drawn.

A better way to chronically reduce calories without feeling hungry or deprived is to eat large amounts of natural foods that have a high nutrient-to-calorie ratio. The Forever Young program suggests that you try to realign your caloric intake by focusing on vegetables and fruits, berries and nuts, water, tea, soymilk, and nonfat dairy. It is also important that you include lean protein with each meal. When you eat this way, you will feel satisfied despite cutting your calorie intake, which will allow you to get and stay fit, lean, and energetic.

A *calorie is* not *a calorie*

It is true that one of the best ways to lose weight and improve your overall health is to simply reduce the number of calories you eat each day. Moreover, losing your excess weight trumps almost anything else you can do to improve your well-being and longevity. Thus, the type of diet you follow might seem to be somewhat irrelevant, as long as it results in weight loss. This is true to some extent, which is why the Atkins diet will improve some health parameters like blood glucose (sugar), triglycerides, and blood pressure. However, the closest you will come to the dietary fountain of youth is to eliminate calories from foods that accelerate aging and consume foods that are loaded with age-defying nutrients. Stick to the good proteins, fats, and carbs prescribed by the Forever Young diet, and you will be thinner, younger, and healthier.

6

STRONG BONES AND A SUNNY DISPOSITION

Joan's mother Kathleen is one of the most impressive women we know. At ninety-two, she remains as bright and curious as ever. She still owns and manages real estate in three states, and she follows the horse racing world like a bookie. For most of her life Kathleen has been decades ahead of her time in both her lifestyle and diet. She embraced the natural whole foods diet in the 1940s and has made a habit of serving fresh vegetables and fruit with every meal. Extra virgin olive oil has been her oil of choice for salads and cooking, and she made lean protein and nuts a staple in the household diet. In short, she figured out and followed the Forever Young diet before we were even born, and so she certainly gets credit for instilling those ideals in Joan's mind—before she ever received any formal training in nutrition. Now in the tenth decade of a remarkably productive and happy life, her health is good except for severe osteoporosis, or weakening of the bones. Her osteoporosis has taken a real toll on her ability to enjoy life, as it has for many American women over age sixty. Her spine has been painfully deformed by multiple compression fractures into a permanent "C" shape so that when she stands, she can only look straight down at her feet. The prevention of osteoporosis has understandably become a passion for Joan.

Fortunately, the knowledge and tools are available today to keep your bones sturdy and resilient so this won't happen to you no matter how long you live. The most effective strategy to prevent or delay osteoporosis involves finding the best of both worlds, and here is the Forever Young program for accomplishing that.

Eight Steps to Lifelong Strong Bones

1. *Vigorous daily exercise.* Cells sense the physical strain on the bones when they are stressed during vigorous activities done while working against gravity. This stimulates hormonal and protein changes that serve to remodel the bone, making it denser and stronger. The skeleton of a female is strongest when she is about twenty to thirty years old. Thereafter, her bone strength often starts to gradually erode. This accelerates at menopause, when the rate of bone loss triples. A study published in the *Archives of Internal Medicine* in May 2004 showed that vigorous exercise in the form of weight lifting twice weekly combined with aerobic exercise two or times weekly prevented the development of osteoporosis after menopause. You can optimize your bone health by staying active. Take the stairs every chance you get, garden, do housework, carry the laundry basket, etc. But you will also need to incorporate weight-bearing exercises like walking, jogging, running, or aerobics, as well as strength-training exercises like weight lifting. And don't think weight lifting is just for men. James tells his women patients over age sixty that if they can do only one exercise, it should be weight lifting. If people stay strong as they age, they will naturally stay more active.

2. *Keep your vitamin D levels high.* A study published in August 2005 in *Current Medical Research and Opinion* found that 98 percent of people admitted for hip fractures were vitamin D deficient. About 90 percent of this vital nutrient is produced by the skin in response to sunlight, so try to get at least ten to fifteen minutes of sunlight daily. However, if you are out in the sun for more than fifteen minutes, wear sunscreen to protect against skin cancer and premature aging of the skin. If you are less than forty years old, take 400 IU of vitamin D daily, and for those who are over forty, shoot for 800 IU daily.

3. *Calcium.* Surprisingly, calcium intake is a relatively poor predictor of who will get osteoporosis. Studies show that the average adult needs about 550 mg of calcium daily to maintain strong bones. Most experts recommend about 1000 mg daily

for men and 1500 mg for women. The real key is not how much calcium you consume, but how much you retain. Your skeleton is in constant flux between bone-building and breakdown. As a youngster your bone-building activity dominated, and thus your bones grew stronger. In midlife, you should be in balance; but by about age thirty to thirty-five, the bone breakdown with loss of skeletal calcium begins to outpace bone building in many people. Thus, it is critical that you stay in calcium balance to keep your bones predominantly in the building process. The other steps in this outline will help to ensure that the calcium you take in will get into your bones and stay there. As with most things, the key is moderation. Too much calcium (more than 2000 mg daily) may increase risk of prostate cancer in men, who are generally less prone to develop osteoporosis than women anyway. We recommend that men take in one or two (but not more) servings of low-fat or fat-free dairy daily.

4. *Maintain proper acid-base balance.* Too much salt, alcohol, caffeine, phosphorus, and protein can leave you in an acidic state. The Forever Young diet emphasizes vegetables and fruits, tea, and water, all of which alkalinize your system and preserve bone strength.

5. *Do not smoke.* Among the many devastating health effects of tobacco is the tendency to turn your strong bones to soft chalk.

6. *Use toothpaste with fluoride and drink tea (which is fluoride-rich).* Fluoride not only keeps your teeth strong, it also helps your bones. If you drink four or more cups of tea per day, your fluoride intake is adequate even without a fluoride toothpaste or fluorinated water.

7. *Make sure you get enough vitamin K.* This vitamin is essential for regulating the blood clotting process, but it also plays a role in bone health. You should be getting 100 micrograms or more daily. Your daily multivitamin should supply about 30 mcgs (micrograms) of vitamin K. To get the remainder, eat nuts and green leafy vegetables regularly—such as spinach, broccoli, brussels sprouts, kale, and dark green lettuce.

8. *Proper posture.* This will help keep your spine and the rest of your musculoskeletal system aligned and minimize abnormal stresses on the bones and joints.

Calcium Sources

Dairy products are the richest source of calcium in our modern diet. Other foods like sardines, vegetables, and nuts, and some mineral waters contain small amounts of calcium as well. However, you would need to consume unrealistically large amounts of vegetables to meet your daily calcium needs. For example, one and one-half cups of cooked kale, two and one-quarter cups of broccoli, or eight cups of cooked spinach supply the same amount of calcium contained in one cup of skim milk.

Nonfat Dairy

Our ancestors got plenty of calcium by eating small bones in fish, birds, and small animals as well as plenty of green leafy vegetables. Today, chewing on bones is considered OK for your dog but definitely unsophisticated for people. So many Americans have an inadequate intake of calcium, which predisposes them to osteoporosis (weak bones) and high blood pressure, among other problems. To make matters worse, we tend to eat too much processed food that makes our systems acidic, as opposed to natural whole foods like fruits and vegetables that alkalinize the system. A chronically acidic system tends to leach calcium out of bones and cause osteoporosis and fractures.

Thus, the dietary keys to strong bones are a variety of fresh produce daily and adequate calcium. If you don't use dairy products, you will probably have to take a supplement or use fortified foods like soymilk to meet your calcium requirement. Dairy is a rich dietary source of calcium, though it is important to choose nonfat or low-fat dairy products to avoid problems like high cholesterol and heart attacks that are associated with eating too much saturated fat. Nonfat dairy products like skim milk are a better choice, and they are also full of high-quality protein, potassium, and vitamin D.

Recent studies show that children and adults who consume nonfat or low-fat milk, yogurt, or cheese (about two to three servings per day) have a lower risk of developing obesity, diabetes, high blood pressure, osteoporosis, and even fractures. It is very difficult to build and maintain strong bones without an adequate intake of calcium. Nonfat milk is satiating due to its high protein and low-calorie nature and may help you attain your ideal weight by hampering fat storage and selectively burning off body fat. If you can drink two (for men) or three (for women) cups of skim milk daily, you will have an easier time losing your excess weight, maintaining an ideal body weight, and building strong bones.

The churning dairy debate

However, dairy products may have a dark side. Epidemiologic studies link high intake of dairy foods to increased risk of ovarian cancer in females and prostate cancer in males, and large long-term studies consistently show no reduction in risk of fracture in those who have a high consumption of dairy. Milk does contain hormones that have been associated with increased risks of malignancy in the prostate.

The traditional goal of 1000 to 1500 mg of calcium daily is probably higher than it needs to be, especially if one is very physically active, has normal vitamin D levels, avoids tobacco, and eats a diet full of vegetables and fruits, and low in salt and alcohol. Under those circumstances the body is able to build and maintain strong bones with a much lower calcium intake—and the European guidelines call for only 700 mg of calcium intake daily. Our ancestors ate no dairy once they were weaned from their mother's milk, and they had no problems maintaining adequate calcium intake due to their active lifestyles, good vitamin D levels from sun exposure, and generous intake of animal and plant foods containing calcium. We believe that an intake of 700 to 1000 mg of calcium daily is probably adequate if you are following the Forever Young program closely.

The Benefits of Soy

The phytochemical antioxidants in soy may help to prevent or delay prostate enlargement and cancer of the prostate. These are just a few of the reasons why soy food is a highly recommended component of the Forever Young program. Soy products are rich in isoflavones, which have been shown to lower blood pressure and cholesterol and may reduce the risks of cardiovascular disease and cancer of the breast and prostate. Incorporate soy into your daily routine by drinking soymilk or eating soy nuts (roasted soybeans) as a snack. If you have blood pressure problems, try to eat the unsalted or lightly salted soy nuts. Men with prostate problems will notice immediate improvements in the frequent nighttime trips to the bathroom if they trade dairy for non–calcium fortified soymilk.

A recent study showed that soy protein is a better choice than high animal protein for people with diabetes and damaged kidneys that are leaking protein into the urine. The study also showed that soy protein raised HDL cholesterol by about 4 percent. In spite of these benefits, we do not recommend more than two servings of soy per day, nor do we think soy phytoestrogens in supplement form are a good idea. The effects of chronically very high levels of these potent plant compounds are still unknown.

Here Comes the Sun

Who hasn't appreciated the feeling of basking in the sun for a few minutes, especially after a stretch of cloudy and cold weather? Amazingly, science now shows us that sunshine has the power to lift our moods, strengthen our bones, and even keep our hearts healthy. No wonder we instinctively enjoy blue-sky sunny days. About 90 percent of the vitamin D in our system is produced by our skin in response to sunlight. Vitamin D is essential for the vitality of every cell and tissue in your body, therefore maintaining normal levels has enormous benefits for overall health. Many Americans have become deficient in this critical nutrient because of our indoor lifestyles. Vitamin D deficiency causes a host of problems like aches and pains in the joints and muscles, osteoporosis and fractures, and possibly even cancer, rheumatoid arthritis, multiple sclerosis (MS), and heart disease. This common nutritional deficiency is easily avoided with modest doses of sunshine and a daily oral dose of vitamin D.

Although too much sun exposure can cause skin cancer and premature aging of the skin, at least ten to fifteen minutes of sunshine per day can help keep your bones and heart healthy. It's just one more reason to make a point of getting outside for some fresh air and daily exercise. If you are out in intense sunlight for more than fifteen minutes, be sure to use sunscreen lotion.

Skin cancers, including potentially lethal melanomas, have been increasing dramatically during the last two or three decades. Sunbathing, tanning salons, and the popularity of the "healthy" tanned look have shouldered the blame for this phenomenon, but in reality we spend less time in the sun than ever. So what is going on? It turns out that how easily you sunburn (a strong risk factor for skin cancer) is strongly influenced by what you eat and drink. When you eat a diet high in calories but low in antioxidants, you are much more likely to get a sunburn. The antioxidants from brightly, deeply pigmented fruits and vegetables, green tea, red wine, onions and garlic, dark chocolate, and soy act as a natural sunscreen, helping to prevent sunburn and possibly skin cancer.

Following the Forever Young program is like applying sunscreen from the inside out—protecting you from skin cancer and aging. The low antioxidant content of the standard American diet may be one of the main reasons that we are seeing a marked increase in the incidence of melanoma and other skin cancers in recent decades, even though we are outside less than we used to be. Additionally, the antioxidant-rich Forever Young diet counteracts the skin-aging effects of the sun by mopping up dangerous free radicals and repairing DNA damage. Finally, our ancestors built a natural tolerance for sun exposure since they were outside every day. You can do this by making a point of getting outside for at least ten to fifteen minutes most days of the week.

7

HOW TO
MAKE IT HAPPEN

Knowing is not enough; we must apply.
Willing is not enough; we must do.

—JOHANN GOETHE

The largest hurdle to overcome in realizing your full potential is the inertia of your comfortable but self-defeating lifestyle. You don't have the energy or will to exercise and eat right in part because your day-to-day routine is robbing you of vitality and enthusiasm. If you can take small steps in the right direction, you can build a self-reinforcing lifestyle that affords you more energy and self-esteem, allowing you to become more active and choose healthier foods and drinks. Nothing succeeds like success. When you make the connection between eating right and feeling better, you will find yourself choosing healthy foods without even having to think about it.

The Secrets of Successful Losers: Change Your Diet Permanently

Experts consider successful weight loss to be losing 10 percent or more of your body weight and keeping it off for one year or more. Even with this relatively modest target, only one in five dieters is successful. Studies indicate there are specific behaviors and attitudes that are common among people who successfully lose weight and keep it off permanently. The National Weight Control Registry tracks about 3,000 "successful losers" who have lost an average of sixty-six pounds and kept it off for five years or more. Another study by Consumer Reports surveyed 32,000 dieters to determine what correlated with successful long-term weight loss. These studies came to similar conclusions: There is no magic bullet, quick fix, or surefire short cut to long-term weight loss. If you are serious about getting rid of the excess baggage for good, you must pay close attention to the tips that follow.

- **Daily exercise.** A program of daily aerobic exercise consistently turns up as the number-one factor in maintaining long-term weight loss. You can lose weight on a diet alone, but you have no chance of keeping it off unless you make exercise a nonnegotiable daily habit, like brushing your teeth. In fact, studies show it takes forty-five to ninety minutes of daily exercise for most previously overweight people to maintain an ideal weight. It doesn't have to be all at once; break it into two or more sessions if you can't find the energy or time to do it in one session. By adding weight training to your exercise routine, you will increase your metabolic rate so that you burn more calories even at rest. Women usually stick with an exercise program if they can do it with one or more friends, while men often do fine working out alone. The antidepressant effects of exercise are a key to reenergizing your life. When you lead a sedentary life you don't have the energy to exercise, creating a vicious cycle that leaves you overweight, depressed, and emotionally drained. The path out of this quagmire is a daily dose of exercise. The more you do it, the more energy you will have, and the more calories you will burn.

- **Shop the "U."** Walk right by the aisles of boxes, cans, and bags full of calorie-dense processed food. When you go to the supermarket, buy nearly all of your food on the U-shaped perimeter of the store. This is where you will find the fresh produce, fresh fish and meats, nonfat dairy, whole-grain bread, water, tea, wine, nuts, berries, etc.

- **Don't think of it as a temporary diet.** This is the eating pattern that will revolutionize and revitalize you if you will continue it for the rest of your life. It will not leave you hungry or irritable. To the contrary, when you start to eat this way, you will feel better, think better, and look better. If you can muster the self-discipline to follow it closely for a few days to weeks, you will stop craving the foods that make you fat and unhealthy like doughnuts and French fries.

- **Do not take days off from your diet.** Days off keep you in the temporary diet mind frame, and binges sabotage your success. People who stay lean permanently do not take days where they allow themselves to eat unlimited amounts of anything they want. One treat usually turns into an excuse to go on a junk-food binge, analogous to the first drink for an alcoholic or the first cigarette for a ex-chain smoker.

- **Rise and shine: Eat breakfast daily.** Eat breakfast to start your day enthused, energetic, and ready to think. This meal should provide almost one-third of your daily intake of calories and protein. When you fill your tank with the right fuel in the morning, you will feel the power throughout the day.

- **One day at a time.** Think of success one step and one bite at a time. The Forever Young program is naturally self-reinforcing; as you follow it, you will begin to feel more energetic, happier, and healthier within hours. You will also be sleeping better and looking better. The short-term benefits of the program will encourage you to stick with it for the long term, and the longer you keep your weight off, the more likely it will be permanent. The threshold seems to be about two years—stay fit and lean for that long, and you will probably be on autopilot after that.

- **Weigh yourself daily or every other day.** Regular feedback is essential for long-term success. You have to see the results of your behavior, whether that be weight gain when you pig-out, or weight loss when you have been eating well. The regular weigh-in is best done first thing in the morning, after you urinate and before you start eating and drinking. Naked is ideal, or weigh-in wearing a minimal amount of clothing that is consistent from one morning to the next.

- **Keep a food diary.** If you find that you are having difficulty making progress in your quest to lose excess body fat, record what you eat. When you conscientiously write down everything you consume, you tend to become more accountable and less likely to cheat or binge.

- **Involve the people in your life in your efforts to become fit and lean.** You will have a better chance of successfully losing weight if you are encouraged and supported in your efforts by family and friends. This is especially true for women, but men are often more successful with a support group as well.

- **Persistence, persistence, persistence.** Remember that neither failure nor success is permanent. Even if you have tried and failed several times before, try again. Successful losers often end up trying all the wrong ways before they finally settle into a no-nonsense plan. Think of your past failures as successes because they highlight methods that will not work for you. When you eliminate the futile strategies and learn from what has and hasn't worked in the past, you will find the way that does work. Tailor a plan that fits your needs, set reasonable goals, and give it your best shot.

- **Tune in to what real hunger is.** Before you put a bite of food in your mouth, make sure you are truly hungry, not just dehydrated and thirsty, or stressed, mad, sad, bored, happy, hurt, or anxious. Additionally, many people feel compelled to eat when someone around them is snacking, regardless of whether they are actually hungry. This kind of mindless overeating will sabotage your weight-loss program and your health. Joan tells her clients they need to have an active ongoing conversation with themselves throughout the day. "Am I really hungry or is this one of those times when I am eating for some other reason?" Come to recognize true hunger, and if you don't feel it, don't eat. If real hunger strikes between meals, choose a healthy snack like nuts, an apple, an orange, or a part-skim mozzarella cheese stick. And if you have just eaten a meal or snack and find yourself craving more food, it may just be emotions, or boredom, or something else besides hunger. So listen closely to your body's cues. It's okay to feel a little hungry—learn to welcome it. Come to recognize that vague gnawing feeling in your belly that signifies real hunger. Imagine that you are feeling this, your body is tapping into your fat stores and melting away the toxic belly fat that ages you and predisposes you to diseases like diabetes and high blood pressure.

- **Do the next right thing.** This program is not an all-or-nothing proposition. If you stray from the diet, think of the next meal as an opportunity to get back on track. Nobody is perfect. Don't focus on a recent poor choice and use it as an excuse to abandon the program, but rather resolve to make the right decision the next time you put something in your mouth.

- **Take responsibility.** This is your life, only you can make it happen. Make taking care of yourself one of your top priorities. This bit of advice sounds selfish on the surface, but it is in fact the best thing you can do for the loved ones in your life and everyone else who relies upon you. The most common excuse we hear about why you can't follow a healthy diet and exercise plan is that you are too busy taking care of everyone else and/or you are consumed with responsibilities at work. No doubt, your life is hectic and overbooked, and unless you make eating right and getting some exercise among your top priorities, they will not happen. Even with good intentions, most people fail because their lives are filled with pressing obligations and distractions. Remember, you owe it to your loved ones to take care of yourself, too.

Emotional Eating: Consumed by Your Feelings

Successful long-term weight control requires you to stop and think before stuffing calories into your mouth. Most people end up with excess body fat because they are mindlessly overeating in response to any number of emotions or situations. Sometimes we eat food to satisfy feelings more than to satiate our hunger. Emotional eating happens when we eat and drink for reasons other than hunger. Emotions like sadness, loneliness, anger, or even happiness often trigger eating like the physical symptom of hunger. There are several distinctions between eating in response to emotions and the true physical craving:

- Emotional cravings appear suddenly; physical hunger comes on gradually.
- When people eat to satisfy an emotional need unrelated to an empty stomach, they often yearn for a specific food like ice cream or chocolate, and only that food will meet the need. In contrast, when you are truly hungry, you are open to any number of foods.
- Emotional hunger demands immediate gratification; physical hunger can usually wait.
- With emotional eating you are more likely to keep eating even after you are full. On the other hand, when you eat because you are truly hungry, you're more likely to stop before overstuffing yourself.
- Emotional eating often leaves you with feelings of guilt and regret after you finish; eating for physical hunger does not.

Ice cream and chocolate are favorite comfort foods for many people, especially women, who also often crave cookies and other sweets. Men seem to be drawn to foods like pizza, steak, and potatoes when emotions compel them to eat. Everybody eats for emotional reasons occasionally, but if you are using eating as the primary strategy for managing your emotions, you are probably going to end up seriously overweight. Hunger is the body's cue that it is low on calories. If you are eating when you aren't hungry, you are likely taking on calories that end up around your midsection as body fat. Experts like Jane Jakubczak, RD, from the University of Maryland have estimated that perhaps 75 percent of overeating in America today is related at least in part to emotions.

How to Deal with Emotional Eating

If you often find yourself hungry, are prone to frequent snacking, or turn to high-calorie comfort foods when emotions bubble up, you need to eat a low-energy-density diet. Our diet is just such a plan—it will fill you up and keep you full longer so emotions cannot derail your efforts to stay lean and healthy. Follow the simple rules of the Forever Young program, and you will be less susceptible to the perils of emotional eating. Here are some pointers to help you avoid emotional eating:

- Pay attention to whether you are looking for food because you are hungry or are you just reflexively eating in response to an emotion like boredom or worry. If you aren't feeling the vague gnawing sensation in the pit of your stomach that signals hunger, do something else instead of putting calories in your mouth.
- Be familiar with emotional eating and figure out what triggers this behavior in you. Some people eat when they are stressed, and others eat when they are happy. Still others eat when they are bored, thirsty, anxious, cold, or almost anything. The "fat and happy" stereotype often applies to twenty-five to forty year olds who tend to overeat when they are contented—after their wedding, following a raise or promotion, during pregnancy, etc.
- When cravings strike and you feel overwhelmed, try getting out for a walk, phoning a friend, lifting weights, cleaning the house, throwing in a load of laundry, even taking a nap or doing some other enjoyable activity to distract you from food. Remove yourself from the vicinity of food. This is another good reason not to keep sweet temptations and junk food around the house.
- If you do feel compelled to eat when you aren't hungry, find a healthy comfort food instead of junk food. For example, an ounce of dark chocolate has redeeming value because of its antioxidant and healthy fat content

(although many chocoholics have a hard time eating just a little chocolate). Better yet, have a cup of unsweetened hot or iced tea, a bottle of water, or a glass of sparkling water with a twist of fresh lime or lemon. Be careful about drinking artificially sweetened soft drinks—these often stimulate cravings for real sweets, the kinds loaded with calories.

- For many people, giving up comfort foods completely is emotionally difficult. But at least try to be moderate when you do give in to the urge to splurge. If you crave unhealthy comfort foods like cheesecake, just have three or four bites and push it away. A few days later you'll still remember it as a pleasurable experience even if you didn't down the whole piece.

Keep in mind that emotional eating tends to occur when you are bored, happy, or sad. Whether you choose a candy bar when you're lonely or a doughnut when you are depressed, understanding how to recognize and control emotional eating is essential to successful weight management for many people.

The Importance of Feedback

Nothing motivates a person like an objective assessment. If you never had to take tests, how hard would you have studied in school? The power of the human psyche to rationalize and deny reality is frightening, but hard numbers are difficult to ignore. They provide an objective bottom line that generally gives you positive feedback when you have been good, and negative feedback when you have gotten distracted and strayed from your healthy routine.

Plan to incorporate regular feedback into your program if you want to succeed in losing excess weight and keeping it off. In her book *Thin for Life*, Ann Fletcher studied "masters of weight loss" (defined as someone who has lost twenty pounds or more and kept it off for at least three years) and found that about 90 percent of them weighed themselves regularly. Joan recommends that her clients weigh themselves at least once weekly. Premenopausal women tend to retain fluid in the days leading up to the start of their period, which is usually reflected in an increased weight of two to four pounds during this phase. This fluid-related weight fluctuation can be a source of frustration if you weigh yourself daily. To minimize inconsistency in the readings, always weigh yourself in the morning, and Saturday is often a good choice because you may not be quite as pressed for time then. It is also important to establish and maintain a buffer zone for your weight. Joan suggests that you set an upper limit of about five pounds above what you consider to be your acceptable weight. Monitor your weight regularly, and if you hit the upper limit, have a strategy ready to implement. This might be intensifying your dietary efforts, exercising more, eliminating sweets and starches altogether for a while, or whatever has worked best for you in the past.

Many women seem to do well in structured programs such as Weight Watchers. In our practice, we utilize the Preventive Cardiology Clinic (PCC) here at the Mid America Heart Institute. James can count on the fact that when his patients get engaged in our PCC, they will almost always do well.

Take Home Messages About Food Labels

If you learn to read a food label, you will have a much better chance of taking home the right foods from the store.

- Don't buy or eat anything with hydrogenated or partially hydrogenated oils (trans fats) in the ingredient list. These are downright toxic, predisposing you to heart disease, cancer, diabetes, and Alzheimer's disease. When you see this on a food label, drop the package, step away from the shelf, and nobody will get hurt.
- Avoid foods and drinks with high fructose corn syrup, sugar, or white flour toward the top of the ingredient list. Think of these as tempting but unnatural fuels that will ruin your looks and your health. Manufacturers are being creative about how to get sugar in products without calling it that on the labels. Stealth forms of sugar to look out for on ingredient lists include: sucrose, honey, pure cane sugar, molasses, corn sweetener, glucose, dextrose, lactose, maltose, fruit juice, and syrup.
- Take a quick glance at the ingredients list. If it is a long list with small print and numerous chemical names, reject the product and move back to the periphery of the store where the natural fresh whole foods are displayed.
- Embrace fiber. When buying bread, purchase only those that list whole-grain flour as the first ingredient. Fiber is your ally, reducing the risks of heart disease and colon cancer and also preventing constipation and diver-

ticulosis. Any grain-based product you consume should have at least three grams of fiber per 100 calories.

- Do not be fooled into thinking processed food items that are advertised as low fat are OK; they are almost always high in calories, sugar, white flour, salt, and other unhealthy ingredients. The same holds for low carb; these are generally unnatural, highly processed foods loaded with toxic substances.

- Avoid artificial sweeteners. These are calorie free, but they may sabotage your weight-loss program nonetheless. Studies show that people who use artificial sweeteners consume more calories during the rest of the day because these unnatural compounds increase your cravings for carbohydrates like sugar and starch.

- Look for the sodium content. Steer clear of anything that has more than 480 mg per serving. Limit your daily intake of sodium to 2300 mg.

- Look at the recommended serving size. The label may say only 100 calories, but if the package contains five servings and you eat the whole bag, you will have consumed 500 calories.

Don't Bring Home the Temptations

Joan always keeps the house stocked with nuts, berries, fruit, vegetables, whole-grain bread, and other healthy snacks. When they are hungry, the kids will *settle* for these healthy snacks, which leave them happy and satisfied. But if you have candy and junk food around, children will often choose these unhealthy options. So don't set yourself and your family up to fail. Keep the junk food out of your home and you will be on your way toward success.

We love ice cream and frozen yogurt, but we generally do not have any of it around the house. About twice a week we go out for an ice cream treat, often riding our bikes, running, or walking a mile or two to get there. We each get one small scoop of ice cream and savor the taste. If we had it at home in unlimited quantities, we would certainly eat more of it, and it would seem like less of a special treat. This way, we get to enjoy ice cream and have a fun excuse to motivate us to get out for an evening workout at the same time.

Burn More Calories Without Even Trying

Fully 60 percent of the calories you burn each day are used for your resting metabolic rate. This is the energy required to just keep the lights on and the furnace running. Activities such as breathing, digesting food, regulating temperature, and keeping your brain thinking and your blood circulating contribute to your resting energy requirements. The resting metabolic rate is highly variable from person to person and accounts for the fact that many people, especially as they age, seem to gain weight even with relatively low-caloric intakes. Losing weight and staying lean are not just a function of how many calories you take in, but also how many calories you burn. Increasing your caloric expenditure through exercise is essential, but you will find it easier to stay lean and fit if you can burn more calories every day without even trying—by cranking up your internal furnace. The Forever Young diet will help you do just that.

Breaking Through Your Set Point Weight

Many scientists who study nutrition and obesity believe that humans have a "set point" or "settling point" for weight. According to this theory, when body weight fluctuates below this set point, powerful involuntary changes in the body and brain try to defend the baseline body weight, especially when calorie intake is reduced. Hunger is one of the obvious mechanisms for restoring weight, but another very important compensation is a downward adjustment in your metabolic furnace. Such changes helped our ancestors survive starvation, but now they only serve to sabotage your efforts to lose your excess fat. Your body senses when the calorie intake drops below what you usually burn in a day, and it automatically goes into starvation mode, dropping your metabolic rate so you burn fewer calories. This phenomenon is obvious to most people who try to lose weight and have some success at first, then notice that they seem to lose little to no more body fat despite an ongoing, marked reduction in calorie intake. Soon their hunger overwhelms their willpower, and they gravitate back to their set point weight. This slowing of the metabolism is often perceptible because you feel fatigued, cold, hungry, and listless. These automatic responses make lasting weight loss beyond the reach for many people. In order to break through this set point and achieve a new lower set point weight, you will have to make the changes in your diet and your lifestyle that are recommended in the Forever Young program.

A fascinating study published in the November 24, 2004, *Journal of the American Medical Association* compared the standard low-fat American Heart Association diet to a low-glycemic-load program like the Forever Young diet. While subjects on both sides of the trial lost weight, those consuming the low-glycemic-load diet did not slow their metabolism down as their weight fell, whereas those consuming more sugar and starch but still losing weight had an 11 percent fall in their resting metabolic rate. This study proves that the best eating style to keep your metabolic rate up is to avoid sugar, starches, and other calorie-dense processed foods. The diet that keeps your metabolic furnace stoked is not low fat or low carb; instead it has a low glycemic load (making it less likely to raise your blood sugar and insulin) and is high in fiber, high in water, and high in good fats with fewer bad fats; it is also moderate to high in protein.

Rev Up Your Metabolism

Here are suggestions that will turn up your idle so you can burn off your stored fuel and feel lean and youthful again.

- Drink green tea. Studies show that people who drink three to four cups of green tea or more per day can increase their metabolic rate by approximately 4 percent, which translates into about six pounds per year.
- Weight training. Muscle tissue is highly metabolically active. At rest, pound for pound, muscle burns nine times more calories than fat tissue. Strength training helps to build muscle, and the more muscle you have on your frame, the faster your basal metabolic rate will be. You should do strength-training exercises at least two to three times per week.
- Get adequate sleep. Sleep deprivation raises stress hormones that can sap your energy and leave you less energetic and less likely to burn calories.
- Add protein to your diet, especially whey protein. A diet that includes adequate amounts of protein will increase your basal metabolic rate. Lean red protein sources increase your basal metabolic rate to a much greater degree than processed carbohydrates like sugar and starch. We recommend shooting for a protein consumption of 20 to 30 percent of your caloric intake. This is easy to accomplish by adding one or two scoops of whey protein to your daily regimen.

- Avoid sugar and other refined carbohydrates. The insulin spike that occurs after carbohydrate consumption lowers your resting metabolic rate. Natural carbohydrates, such as those found in vegetables, fruits, and whole grains, will provide energy without resulting in a surge of insulin. Grapefruit in particular seems to be able to increase your metabolism and is an ideal food to eat daily if you want to become leaner and healthier.
- Drink at least one liter of water daily. Just adding water to the diet increases your metabolism and helps with weight loss.
- Eat breakfast. The combination of healthy carbs, lean protein, and water or tea at breakfast is a surefire way to start strong and stay focused and energetic throughout your day.
- Exercise more frequently. Your metabolism remains elevated for one to two hours following every workout. If you do not have time for a big, complicated workout at your favorite gym, simply take twenty minutes to go for a brisk walk, climb stairs, or lift a few weights. But remember, it is almost impossible to exercise off substantial amounts of body fat with activity alone—it takes thirty-five miles of running or walking to burn the 3,500 calories that one pound of body fat contains. Exercise must be combined with a prudent diet.

Size Matters

We hear many people complain that they eat a healthy diet but still pack on pounds. On a daily basis, the average American adult is now burning about 200 calories less and taking in an extra 350 extra calories per day compared to thirty years ago. Consider that if every day you consistently consume just 100 calories more than you burn, in one year you will gain about ten pounds of body fat. Even if you are reasonably conscientious about what you eat, you are destined to get fat if you do not also pay attention to how much you eat and how much exercise you are getting. To make matters worse, the food industry is conspiring to fool us into overconsuming food at every opportunity.

The fast-food industry pioneered portion distortion starting about twenty years ago when they discovered it was a successful ploy for increasing their business. Now, most Americans are clueless about appropriate portion sizes. We must relearn what a proper serving is for various foods, and then be disciplined about our eating habits. Your stomach is about the size of your two fists. You can ignore portion control when it comes to most vegetables. The goal is to fill up your stomach with low-calorie, highly nutritious vegetables and fruits that will limit the amount of room left in there for the high-calorie foods. Lean protein like turkey, chicken, fish, or lean red meat is an essential element of each meal but should be limited to about the size of a deck of cards or the palm of your hand. If you feel compelled to eat mashed potatoes, rice, or other starches, limit the amount to one-half cup—about the size of a computer mouse. Rich desserts like cheesecake, pies, and ice cream should be limited to only a few (not more than four) bites.

Portion control is one of the critical issues in long-term successful weight loss. You will have to develop a consistent internal guide to not just what, but also how much you eat. Dr. Barbara Rolls, author of *The Volumetrics Weight-Control Plan*, has championed the cause of portion control for the past several years. Americans spend more that $33 billion on weight-loss products and services, but the simple, basic, undeniable truth is that in order to lose weight you will have to eat fewer calories and exercise more. Taking diet pills or diuretics, using weight-loss supplements and countless other "guaranteed, proven methods to magically cause your excess fat tissue to melt away," are virtually always ineffective over the long term, usually expensive, and sometimes even dangerous. The good news is that you can get your weight back under control by focusing on portion control, rather than willpower alone, which on its own is destined to fail almost every time.

Portion Control Induces Weight Loss

A recent study published in the September 9, 2004, issue of *Obesity Research* found that overweight individuals who focused their efforts in controlling the portion sizes of what they ate were more successful in losing weight and keeping it off than people using other strategies. Although an increase in daily exercise also helped people drop excess pounds, the investigators found that a portion control strategy had the best results.

After two years of follow-up, investigators found that those individuals who actively controlled portion size were more likely to lose weight. About 38 percent of the obese people who practiced food portion control *lost* 5 percent or more of their body weight, and in contrast, 33 percent of the participants who did not consistently practice portion control *gained* 5 percent or more of their body weight. Practicing the other strategies also improved the odds of losing weight, but portion-size control had the greatest impact.

You can bring your daily calorie balance back into line with a few simple substitutions. Sugars add calories that are devoid of vitamins, minerals, or fiber. These empty calories cause aging and obesity, and you need to eliminate them. You can save about 150 calories by drinking water instead of a single high fructose sweetened soda. You can shave 190 calories from your daily intake by snacking on a small piece of fruit rather than a candy bar. You can reduce your calorie intake by 140 to 280 calories by eating smaller, more sensible portions of your favorite foods.

Sensible serving sizes:
> Postage stamp = one teaspoon of butter or margarine
> Deck of cards = three ounces of meat
> Ping-pong ball = two tablespoons of peanut butter
> Pair of dice = one ounce of cheese

How to Keep Your Portion Sizes Down

Follow these tips for reducing portion size and shedding excess body fat:

- Healthy high-calorie foods like nuts and berries and sweet fruits like bananas and watermelon should be limited in quantities unless you are an athlete burning thousands of calories daily with vigorous exercise. A handful is about the right serving size for nuts. Berries should be limited to about one-half cup daily. If you are trying to lose weight, bananas should be generally limited to only one every other day, or a half banana daily. You can eat all the broccoli, spinach, bell peppers, grapefruit, apples, carrots, asparagus, nonstarchy vegetables or less-sweet fruit you want. In fact, the more of these foods the better: They will fill you up and load your system with antiaging disease-fighting phytonutrients but add relatively few calories.

- Pay attention to serving size when you dine out. Most restaurants serve meals that are about twice as large as we need.

- Limit the amount of meals eaten at fast-food restaurants. If you do eat at fast-food joints, order water or tea and a salad with grilled not fried meat. Use only one-half of a packet of salad dressing or choose a low-fat vinaigrette.

- When having a treat such as chocolate, movie-theater popcorn, or a cookie, always choose the smallest serving. Your instinct is to finish the whole thing, no matter what size.
- Whole-grain products are the only foods made from grain you should be eating, and you should have one to three servings per day, such as a slice of whole-grain bread with peanut butter for breakfast. Or if you prefer a sandwich, make it open faced or folded over. Oatmeal is another great choice for your whole grain—get the old-fashioned or steel-cut oats. These varieties are less processed and higher in fiber and thus slower to digest. Eat oats raw if you can, as this really slows the digestion process.
- If you decide to have an occasional high-calorie sweet or rich beverage, pour it into a tall thin glass and use plenty of ice. This will limit the portion size but still fool you into thinking you are getting a large drink.
- Most people underestimate their food intake by at least a third. Learn how many calories are in different foods and change your habits accordingly. Skip "value meals" and "economy-sized" servings of fast food or munchies. Share your food with friends and family. Remember, less is more when it comes to calories.
- Eat protein three times per day, but limit the amount to a piece of meat, chicken, or fish about the size and thickness of the palm of your hand or a deck of cards.

Fewer Food Choices: The Answer to Your Weight Problem?

Having too many food choices, especially of bad foods, appears to play a real role in the expanding American waistline. Some studies show that the average adult has increased his or her caloric intake by as much as 350 calories per day over the past three decades. During this same period, the number of food choices has skyrocketed, and most of them are synthetic high-calorie options that taste great but predispose you to problems like obesity, aging, and disease. The more varied your diet, the more calories you consume, but by limiting the variety of available foods in your immediate environment you can decrease your intake of calories. Psychologists call this technique stimulus control. Keeping cigarettes and ashtrays away from smokers who are trying to quit improves their success rates. Keeping the bad foods out of your cupboards and refrigerator will improve your chances of making the right choices when you are hungry at home.

Apparently, it's not just humans who find that variety makes foods irresistible. Dozens of studies in recent years show that you can induce animals to eat more by simply giving them more variety without increasing the total amount of calories available. Now there are nine studies in humans showing that more food choices usually mean more calories consumed, even when the food choices are seemingly unimportant. For example, researchers in one study found that people ate 14 percent more per meal when they were offered two different shapes of pasta rather than one. In 2001, Researchers from the University of Buffalo verified this trial by analyzing thirty-nine different animal and human trials that all came to the same conclusion: More food choices compel us to eat more.

The variety effect in humans and other mammals is partially explained by the fact that we seem to prefer food that differs from what we just ate. So it is clear that fewer choices in food on a day-to-day basis would be helpful in keeping weight under control. How to make this happen is a more problematic issue. One effective way to reduce variety is to consider major types of foods—for example, highly processed ones and those containing trans fats, HFCS, sugar, or white flour—should be off-limits. If you can discipline yourself to think this way, you will automatically eliminate the majority of foods, particularly the unhealthy ones that you are likely to have access to in your daily routine.

Eating Out Without Pigging Out

Americans are eating more and more meals away from home. You must be careful not to sabotage your weight-management plan when you eat out, so here are a few important tips to help you dine sensibly away from home:

1. *Do not show up at the restaurant famished. Eat a piece of fruit or a drink a large glass of water before leaving for dinner.*
2. *Start drinking water or tea when you sit down at the restaurant.*
3. *Tell the waiter not to bring bread to your table.*
4. *Choose foods that are baked, broiled, boiled, poached, steamed, grilled, roasted, or stir-fried.*
5. *Ask that dressings, sauces, and spreads be served on the side and use these sparingly.*
6. *Trim off visible fat; remove skin from poultry.*
7. *Limit alcohol to one or two drinks. Alcoholic drinks are high in calories.*
8. *Skip dessert or share an order with one or more other people at the table. Our favorite dessert is fresh berries with a little milk or cream on the side.*
9. *Avoid menu items that are fried or breaded or are prepared with cheese, cream, or butter.*
10. *Ask for smaller portions or have half boxed in advance for you to bring home.*
11. *Share your meal—order one dinner and have the waiter bring it on two plates.*

8

NUTRITIONAL SUPPLEMENTS

No supplement will make up for a poor diet and a sedentary lifestyle—don't kid yourself into thinking otherwise. Many people become distracted by taking handfuls of various supplements on a daily basis, and tend to be lulled into a false sense of security by believing outlandish claims about their effectiveness. Although most of these compounds are harmless, they are expensive and sometimes are counterproductive with respect to your health. We strongly suggest that you get most of your essential nutrients and antioxidants from food—not supplements. Most diet books are filled with chapters about various supplements and their potential benefits, but you won't find that here. There is only one way to get the optimal amount of nutrients in your diet, and that is the old-fashioned way—you have to eat them. We suggest that most of you take only a standard multivitamin, an omega-3 supplement, and whey protein. Some people may also need to take glucosamine/chondroitin.

Studies by Loren Cordain, PhD, and others indicate that hunter-gatherers typically obtained approximately half to two-thirds of their calories from animal sources—mostly in the form of lean, freshly killed wild game. They also consumed everything edible on the carcass, including cartilage and marrow. This ensured that they were eating a diet high in branched chain amino acids (the proteins that are best for building and repairing tissue), omega-3 fats, and glucosamine/chondroitin (the proteins used to make and repair cartilage). Although most of us today are eating plenty of meat, it has a very different nutritional profile–higher in saturated fats, lower in protein, and devoid of omega-3 fats and cartilage. It is no coincidence that three of the supplements we recommend—omega-3 fats, whey protein, and glucosamine/chondroitin—all are replacing nutrients that were present in our natural diet but deficient in the modern diet. Many people need to a supplement to provide their bodies with these critically important compounds that are needed to achieve optimal health.

Multivitamins—Nutritional Insurance

A good multivitamin provides approximately 100 percent of the recommended daily allowance for major nutrients such as essential vitamins and minerals. If you closely follow the Forever Young program, you will be getting generous quantities of virtually all the major nutrients. Since you may not eat an ideal diet every day, take a multivitamin for insurance—to cover any potential shortcomings your diet may have. Make sure your multivitamin has at least 400 units of vitamin D. It is best to avoid multivitamins with iron unless you are a female who is still having regular periods or you are known to be iron deficient. Also, be sure to avoid supplements that have more than 10,000 units of vitamin A and/or beta-carotene. We do not recommend single nutrient supplements like high-dose vitamin C, vitamin E, folic acid or beta-carotene. Well-designed scientific trials have consistently reported no benefit and sometimes even some harm from these supplements. For instance, a study from the August 2005 issue of the journal *Alzheimer's and Dementia* found that people with the highest intake of folate (found in foods like avocados and leafy greens) in their diet had the lowest risk of developing Alzheimer's disease. In contrast, the Norwegian Vitamin Trial presented at the European Society of Cardiology Congress in September 2005 found that a daily supplement containing 800 mcg folic acid (the synthetic form of folate used in vitamins) slightly increased the risk of having a heart attack or stroke among 3,749 people during a 3.5 year follow-up period after an initial heart attack.

The best way to get extra nutrients is to eat a highly nutritious diet of fresh whole foods. For instance, if you are impressed with the benefits of vitamin C, take a multivitamin with the standard daily value of this nutrient, but also eat generous quantities of fruits and vegetables that are especially rich in C, such as citrus fruits (but not juices), kiwi, and broccoli.

Omega-3 Fatty Acids: the Most Important Supplement

Why does Sea World have a seafood restaurant?? I'm halfway through my fish burger and I realize, Oh my God. . . . I could be eating a slow learner.
—LYNDA MONTGOMERY

A sharper mind, a happier mood, a healthier heart, a leaner body, and less inflammation: Thousands of scientific studies have documented an astounding array for physical, mental, and emotional benefits conferred by omega-3 supplementation. Omega-3 fats nourish the cells of the skin, hair, nerves, brain, heart, and virtually all of the tissues and organs. You are what you eat. This overused cliché is literally true when we are talking about the type of fats we consume. The membranes of the cells throughout your body are mostly composed of lipids (fats). Omega-3 fats were plentiful in our natural food chain. Countless generations before us ate a high omega-3 diet of wild game, leafy greens, nuts, and especially fish. Unfortunately modern food manufacturers have squeezed the omega-3s out of our diet and replaced them with harmful saturated and trans fats.

Salmon swimming in the frigid waters of the Arctic Ocean are perfectly soft and supple even though their body temperature is just a few degrees above freezing because the lipids in their cell membranes are mostly omega-3 fats. These fats remain liquid even down to temperatures below the freezing point of water (32 degrees Fahrenheit). Imagine you raised these fish in a warm farm pond in Florida and fed them nothing but French fries, stick margarine, doughnuts, and other foods high in trans fats. If you then transported them to the Arctic, upon release they would be transformed to the rigid consistency of a stick of margarine floating in ice water.

The melting point of trans fats and saturated fats are much higher and thus they are solid at room temperature. When you eat a diet high in these lipids your cell membranes become stiff and dysfunctional. You may not notice the hardening as dramatically as the salmon in our story because you have the advantage of being warm-blooded. But the type of fat incorporated into your cell membranes profoundly affects your tissues, especially the electrically sensitive ones like your brain, eyes, and heart. If you want your tissues to remain soft, supple, responsive, and youthful, you must provide them with the preferred fats to incorporate into their cell membranes.

The rigid trans fats and saturated fats predispose us to inflammation, dementia, heart attack, diabetes, and cancer. Omega-3 and monounsaturated fats like those found in fish, nuts, avocados, and olive oil protect against these problems. They also reduce the generalized inflammation in joints and other tissues. One study even reported a lower risk of erectile dysfunction in males consuming higher quantities of omega-3 fat.

My colleague and close friend William Harris, PhD, is a pioneer and foremost authority on omega-3 fats. He has done research showing that the omega-3 content of the cells in your body is by far the most accurate blood test for predicting who will die suddenly of cardiac arrest, which causes 20 percent of all deaths and is still the most common cause of mortality in America. He has also shown that getting the level of omega-3 fatty acids in your cell membranes into a healthy range is usually accomplished by taking two or three capsules per day of an omega-3 (fish oil) supplement. This has been proven in large randomized studies to cut the risk of sudden cardiac death in heart attack survivors by half.

The Omega Effect

Among the possible benefits of a daily omega-3 supplement are improved brain function. The tissue of the brain is made up of over 60 percent fat. In humans, eating our natural diet, much of the structural fat in the brain is in the form of DHA (docosahexaenoic acid) the most important omega-3 fat. The DHA level in the brain is normally fivefold higher than in the blood. We refer to the mood-raising, brain-boosting abilities of omega-3 fats as *the omega effect*. When you supplement your diet with fish oil, especially one that is rich in DHA, you may notice a happier, more optimistic and focused outlook. The omega effect is often discernable to us in our own mental functioning, as well as in our family, friends, coworkers, and patients.

Over the past 100 years we have seen a marked increase in the occurrence of major depression—and an earlier onset of this disease. It is no coincidence that during this same time there have been striking changes in the type of fats consumed. The countries with the highest intake of fish have the lowest rates of depression.

Only one in 833 Japanese people are depressed, and they consume a large amount of omega-3 fats. In contrast, the people of North America have one of the lowest intakes of omega-3 in the world, and the incidence of depression is 50 times higher than the Japanese. Some but not all randomized placebo-controlled trials have demonstrated that omega-3 supplementation may improve depression. Omega-3 appears to normalize the levels of neurotransmitters (brain chemicals), which can help to brighten your mood.

Eating fish five times weekly reduced stroke by 31 percent according to a study published in the July 2004 issue of the journal *Stroke*. These investigators found that eating oily fish like salmon even once a week reduced stroke by about 13 percent. The omega-3 fats also protect your brain against Alzheimer's disease and other forms of dementia. A report from the July 2003 issue of the journal *Archives of Neurology* found that people who ate fish more than once a week had a 60 percent lower risk of Alzheimer's disease compared to those who rarely or never ate fish. Upon further investigation, these researchers determined that DHA was the specific omega-3 that played the most important role in preventing dementia.

More Good News About Omega-3

Omega-3 oils also reduce inflammation throughout the body. A study from the University of Florida showed that a combination of omega-3, flavonoids, and vitamin E helped speed the healing process in sore muscles after long runs or intense weight-lifting sessions. In a two-week study, the men who took a supplement of these nutrients had 50 percent less inflammation in their muscles compared to those who took a placebo. The anti-inflammatory effect of omega-3 may also account in part for the decreases in arthritis, asthma, inflammatory bowel disease, and possibly colon, prostate, and breast cancers noted in some studies in people who eat a diet rich in these fats.

A recently published placebo-controlled trial in twenty-seven women with lupus found that omega-3 supplementation significantly improved their symptoms. Lupus is a serious autoimmune disease caused by excessive and inappropriate inflammation throughout the body. Additionally, omega-3 is one of our best therapies for normalizing high triglyceride levels. High-dose omega-3 (two to five grams of EPA + DHA per day) will lower these bad blood lipid levels by 20 to 50 percent and raise the good cholesterol (HDL) level by about 8 percent.

> You know why fish are so thin? They eat fish.
> —JERRY SEINFELD

Intake of fish and omega-3 fats can also help to restore and maintain normal weight. A recent study showed a 7 to 14 percent increase in fat burning during exercise in people who received a fish oil supplement for about three to five weeks. Other studies show that fish consumption improves the level of leptin, a hormone related to appetite. The lean protein in fish also results in improved satiety, leading to fewer cravings for snacks and less overeating.

Bringing Your Omega-3 Levels Back to Normal

Those who are skeptical about omega-3 like to remind us about what they used to say about snake oil: "It's good for whatever ails you." However, the fact that most of us are eating an omega-3-deficient diet is precisely why this supplement has shown such wide-ranging impressive benefits in scientific trials. When you take most other supplements like vitamins E, C, or A, for example, you are usually bringing your already normal levels into above-normal ranges. Supplementing an already normal level to a supernormal level may result in minor benefits for some conditions, but it can also worsen health when megadoses are used. Bringing a depressed level of an essential nutrient back into a normal range is an entirely different kettle of fish. When the scurvy-afflicted seventeenth-century British sailors were given limes to replenish their deficient vitamin C levels, all of their complaints miraculously improved. Their gums stopped bleeding, their skin improved, their joints became healthy again, and they stopped dying. Similarly, if you are deficient in omega-3 (as 90 percent of Americans are), many diffuse complaints like depression, achy joints, failing memory, rashes, fatigue, and palpitations may improve when you take an omega-3 supplement and bring your levels back into a normal range.

How much omega-3 do you need?

According to the USDA guidelines, Americans should strive for about 500 mg of DHA plus EPA per day. These two essential fatty acids are found mainly in fish. In order to meet these requirements, an individual must consume at least two oily fish meals per week or use omega-3 fish oil supplements. Since 2002, the American Heart Association has recommended the same dosage for healthy individuals, but

1000 mg daily for those with known heart disease. The USDA diet guidelines also acknowledge the research indicating omega-3's impact on improved heart and brain functioning as well as other benefits to the body.

You should try to eat fish two to three times weekly, avoiding fried fish and large carnivorous species like shark, swordfish, and fish caught in contaminated waters like most freshwater lakes in America. These fish can contain dangerous contaminants like mercury or pesticides, especially in their skin. To avoid consuming these, remove and discard the fish skin, visible fat, and dark flesh before cooking. The best choice for cooking fish is to broil, grill, bake, or boil rather than fry.

Cod liver oil can contain toxic residues such as PCBs, dioxin, and mercury. However, a study published in the January 2005 issue of *Archives of Pathology and Laboratory Medicine* evaluated five brands of over-the-counter standard fish oil capsules for toxic residue content. None of the five brands studied contained detectable amounts of environmental toxins such as PCBs, and pesticides like DDT and organochlorines. In a previous report, the same group of scientists found that the mercury content of standard fish oil capsules was below the detectable limit. The FDA designates up to three grams daily of omega-3 as "Generally Recognized as Safe"—its safest label.

Some people complain of a fishy aftertaste or belching after taking fish oil. This is the only real side effect of fish oil and can be minimized by using a more highly concentrated "pharmaceutical-grade" omega-3 supplement, keeping the bottle in the freezer, or using an enteric coated variety.

We believe the evidence indicates a more optimal dose of omega-3 to be about 1000 to 1500 mg of DHA + EPA daily. To accomplish this you will need to consume about 2000 to 3000 mg of highly purified fish oil (usually about 50 percent DHA + EPA) per day, or three to five 1000 mg capsules of standard fish oil (generally about 30 percent DHA + EPA) like those found at your neighborhood pharmacy. The capsules can be taken all at one time, generally with a meal, or in two divided doses, such as with breakfast and the evening meal.

For all its benefits, omega-3 fat does have one downside—it is easily oxidized and thus in high doses can deplete your body's antioxidant levels. To prevent this you should try to use extra virgin olive oil as your primary cooking and salad oil. Extra virgin olive oil is rich in antioxidants, including vitamin E and squalene, which provide protection against oxidation of the omega-3 fat, ensuring that you will get the full benefits without any downside from fish oil supplementation. If you have triglyceride levels over 150 mg/dL, you may need 2000 to 5000 mg of EPA + DHA to normalize your triglycerides and risk of heart disease.

How Much Omega-3 Are You Getting?

Look at the label. The amount of fish oil is not the important number—it is the amount of EPA and DHA, the protective omega-3 fats. What you are interested in is the amount of EPA and DHA per serving. Add up the amount of EPA + DHA and figure out how many capsules you will have to take to come up with at least 1000 mg per day.

Toxic Contaminants: The Dark Side of Fish

In recent years, PCB (a pesticide) contamination of farmed salmon has been highlighted in the press. This contaminant is ubiquitous in domestic meat, fish, and dairy foods. The levels in farmed salmon are modest and overshadowed by the tremendous and proven benefits of the omega-3 and other nutrients in this delicious protein source. Scientists estimate that if you were to eat four ounces of salmon twice weekly for seventy years, you might increase your risk of cancer due to PCB exposure by as much as one in 100,000—a trivial and essentially meaningless risk. On the other hand, two fatty fish meals per week reduces your risk of dying of sudden cardiac death, the single most common cause of death in our society, by about 50 percent.

"Friends don't let friends eat farmed salmon" is a bumper sticker you may have seen recently. This widely held misconception that farmed salmon contains far more toxic contaminants than wild salmon is based on a study by Ronald A. Hites and others that appeared in the journal *Science* in January 2004. Subsequent expert analyses concluded that Hites was on very thin ice in making the recommendation that people avoid farmed salmon. In the spring 2004 issue of *Eating Well*, Steven Malloy stated, "Junk science doesn't get much fishier than the recent scary headlines about farmed salmon being a cancer risk. In fact, there has never been a single (adverse) health effect associated with consumption of farmed salmon despite countless people eating millions of tons of it over the past twenty years. That's no surprise since PCBs, dioxins, and other so-called contaminants considered in the study have never been scientifically shown to cause harm in humans at the typical exposure levels."

In addition, these analyses have shown that the levels of PCBs in wild salmon are about as high as those in the farmed fish. And all of these levels are very low and in line with those found in domestic beef, poultry, and dairy. So forget about the myth that farmed salmon is a health risk. Eating omega-3-rich fish like wild or farmed salmon is one of your best bets for staying healthy and youthful in the long term. Dermatologist Dr. Nicholas Perricone believes salmon is among the healthiest protein sources because in addition to the high levels of omega-3, it contains DMAE. This is a human neurochemical that has been shown to reduce wrinkle formation by improving facial muscle tone. Also, the orange pigment in wild salmon is astaxanthin, which is a powerful anti-inflammatory antioxidant.

A more realistic concern is mercury contamination. The table on page 138 outlines the safe and unsafe varieties of fish. We recommend that most people eat safe fish two to four times per week and take a daily supplement of omega-3 oil to be sure they have plenty of these fats that are critical for keeping heart and brain healthy and happy.

Avoiding Mercury

Methylmercury is a highly toxic compound that is present in some types of fish. The FDA and other health authorities are strongly warning pregnant women and children to avoid certain types of fish to reduce intake of methylmercury. A high intake of mercury has been documented to cause impairment of vision and damage the central nervous system, causing seizures, brain dysfunction, and even birth defects. Intake of toxic quantities of mercury was a large problem in the past, especially in some professions that utilized mercury compounds directly (hence the term "mad as a hatter"). Mercury poisoning from fish is a much rarer disorder, but still one to be considered.

Dr. Charles Santerre from Purdue University has released clear guidelines about safe consumption of fish and seafood. These are relevant to pregnant and nursing women, women who expect to become pregnant, and children under fifteen years of age. Other cautious consumers may wish to reduce their intake along these lines, as well. If you eat fish and seafood frequently, you can have your blood tested for mercury to see if this is an issue you should be concerned about. If the level is elevated, simply restrict your intake of the fish listed below. Note, however, that tea consumption seems to lower mercury levels. A recent study of Canadians with a high fish intake found that those who drank tea frequently had the lowest blood mercury levels. The University of Quebec researchers speculated that the tea flavonoids may bind with heavy metals and escort them out of the body. If you limit your fish intake, be sure to take a daily pharmaceutical-grade omega-3 supplement to be sure you are getting adequate amounts of this vitally important nutrient.

Never Eat **(high mercury level):**	king mackerel, shark, swordfish, marlin, tile fish (also known as golden bass or golden snapper)
One Meal per Month **(moderate mercury level):**	bluefish, croaker, orange roughy, pollock, grouper, halibut, northern lobster, marlin, moonfish, red snapper, sablefish, saltwater bass, wild trout, tuna steaks
One Meal per Week **(low mercury level):**	Cod, crab, haddock, herring, lobster (spiny), mahimahi, tuna (canned white), whitefish
No Limit **(lowest mercury level):**	salmon, scallops, shrimp, sole, tilapia, farmed rainbow trout, tuna (canned, light, and farmed yellow fin), farmed catfish, clams, crayfish, flounder, oysters, perch (saltwater and freshwater)

Source: Indiana Fishing Advisory (http://fn.cfs.purdue.edulanglingindiana)

Developed with the Family Nutrition Program, by Charles Santerre, PhD

Whey Protein

We strongly recommend whey protein as a staple in your diet. This is one of the key Forever Young antiaging recommendations. Whey protein is a source of pure, natural dairy amino acids that make up about 20 percent of the protein in milk and is one of the highest quality proteins you can consume. It is found in the whitish translucent liquid that is separated from milk during the cheese-making process. Despite the fact that whey is derived from dairy, it will not cause problems for lactose-intolerant people because the protein is isolated and purified, leaving behind the sugars (lactose) as well as other undesirables like saturated fat.

Protein is the best nutrient for producing satiety (the sensation of being full), and also helps build muscle and keeps your metabolic furnace cranked up–giving you more energy while burning off more calories. You are designed to thrive best on a diet rich in high-quality protein, but the protein our ancestors ate was lean, higher in omega-3 fats, low in saturated fat, and devoid of dangerous chemicals like nitrites, industrial pollutants, synthetic hormones, herbicides, pesticides, preservatives, and added salt. Furthermore, most of their protein was eaten raw. Although cooking meat and fish is great for killing microbes and parasites (not to mention improving the flavor), the high temperatures can denature the proteins and fats, creating dangerous carcinogens like heterocyclic amines.

Whey protein is an ideal and clean source of high-quality protein in a convenient form that is completely free of any of these contaminants or carcinogens, while many other protein sources are not. For example, too much fatty red meat can increase cardiac risk factors, and if the meat is charred and overdone, over the years it may increase risk of cancer as well. Fish is ideal for many reasons, but some species are often contaminated by mercury and pesticides, and some people do not prefer the taste of fish.

Whey protein is a natural, safe, and neutral-tasting protein source that will give you the best of both worlds. If you use a clean and pure whey protein product, you will get the benefits of a high-quality protein rich in branched chain amino acids that will help you to achieve your ideal body weight, improve your immunity, boost your antioxidant antiaging defenses, and keep you filled up.

Exercise temporarily alters the gene function in your muscles, making them more receptive to incorporating amino acids from a protein meal. Our ancestors usually found themselves eating animal protein after vigorous exertion, such as the typical effort required to track and kill a wild animal. Within an hour or two after strenuous physical exercise, the body anticipates that protein is likely to be consumed, thus making available the essential building blocks for growing stronger muscle and connective tissue and repairing damage. Whey is a biologically complete protein great for building and repairing muscle. To become stronger and leaner, consume whey protein within one to two hours of an exercise session—especially one that involved strength training.

Whey isolate, however, should not be your primary protein source. Meat, fish, dairy, and eggs all provide high-quality protein and contain additional nutrients as well. Red meat is high in vitamin B_{12}, iron, and zinc. Fish is the primary source of omega-3 fats. Dairy is a source of calcium, and egg yolks contain lutein, an important carotenoid antioxidant that helps to protect your eyes and heart. Consider whey as the main protein source at one meal (breakfast, for example) and/or for a snack during the day, but use different protein sources at other meals. Whey powder is fast and easy to use—just stir a scoop into water or a beverage, such as skim milk or soymilk.

The Benefits of Whey

Even during the Italian Renaissance in the 1500s, people realized the health benefits of whey. Two prevalent sayings were, "If everyone were raised on whey, doctors would be bankrupt," and "If you want to live a healthy and active life, drink whey and dine early." Whey protein confers eight distinct benefits that will help you recapture the appearance and vitality of your youth.

1. Whey contains a high level of cysteine, an essential amino acid that stimulates the body's antioxidant production and thus bolsters the immune system and neutralizes free radicals that promote aging, heart disease, and cancer.
2. Whey helps to build muscle protein better than any other source because it is uniquely rich in all the essential amino acids.
3. Whey protein burns fat, especially inside your abdomen, where it is the most unattractive and the most dangerous for your health.
4. Whey increases satiety, thereby lowering your daily intake of calories and helping to prevent aging and disease as well as promoting weight loss.

5. When substituted for other protein sources, whey reduces the load of toxic proaging and potentially carcinogenic substances found in meat, fish, and poultry.

6. Whey protein may reduce depression and emotional stress because it is high in tryptophan—an amino acid that improves mood and sleep quality in some individuals.

7. Whey protein, when added to a high-carbohydrate meal, blunts the spike in blood sugar seen in both healthy and diabetic individuals, as reported in the July 2005 issue of the *American Journal of Clinical Nutrition*.

8. The amino acids in whey protein are exactly the building blocks your body needs to restore the youthful luster and fullness to your hair and give you smooth, shiny, and strong nails. You may notice an improvement in the appearance and strength of your hair and nails when you use whey protein on a daily basis.

How to Choose a High-Quality Whey Product

Look for whey protein isolate, which is a more highly purified form of whey. This will enable quick and easy digestion of the essential amino acids needed by the body for healthy and strong muscles, skin, hair, and nails. Whey protein is best bought in large containers (two to five pounds), since it needs to be consumed regularly to reap the health benefits. We suggest a dose of about twenty to twenty-five grams daily, which is usually about one scoop per day. The whey product should have less than 150 mg of sodium per serving and be sugar free. Look for a whey powder that contains not more than a few other ingredients besides whey protein isolate.

Glucosamine and Chondroitin

You awaken in the morning and begin to notice a slightly swollen and sore knee, with generalized aches in your back—enough to discourage you from taking the stairs and causing you to lose interest in your daily walk. So begins the relentless downward spiral of arthritis: inactivity and weight gain, leading to worsening joint inflammation, and ultimately immobility. Osteoarthritis—wear-and-tear arthritis or degenerative joint disease—has become so common as to be the norm for middle-aged and older Americans. Even though arthritis is not a life-threatening disease, it can seriously impair your quality of life by leaving you in constant pain and limiting your active lifestyle.

The standard treatment for osteoarthritis is one of the NSAIDs (nonsteroidal anti-inflammatory drugs), such as ibuprofen or naproxen. These drugs can reduce arthritis pain for a few hours but only mask the symptoms—if anything they worsen the long-term joint health. Additionally, NSAIDs are dangerous drugs, accounting for 16,500 deaths and over 100,000 hospitalizations annually in the United States (mostly due to bleeding from the stomach or intestines).

A much safer and more effective approach to the treatment of arthritis is combination therapy with the over-the-counter natural substances glucosamine and chondroitin. In osteoarthritis the cartilage becomes inflamed and is gradually eroded away, eventually destroying the padding in the joint and leaving bone grinding against bone. Chondroitin sulfate is a major constituent of cartilage, tendons, and ligaments, where it provides structure, holds water and nutrients, and allows other important molecules like oxygen to diffuse into the joints (which is important as cartilage has no direct supply of blood). A chondroitin supplement provides unique nutrients that nourish and lubricate the joints.

Glucosamine is another naturally occurring substance in your body, and is important in the formation and repair of articular (joint) cartilage. A large and growing body of scientific data suggests that glucosamine and chondroitin are effective at improving arthritic pain and slowing cartilage erosion and joint destruction. In 2000, Dr. T. McAlindon, MD, published a meta-analysis in the *Journal of the American Medical Association* that evaluated these trials in composite and concluded that chondroitin showed a large benefit and glucosamine a moderate benefit in the treatment of osteoarthritis. These supplements are even more effective when used in combination. If you tend to be skeptical of scientific studies, try using glucosamine and chondroitin on your aging arthritic dog for a few weeks and see how much easier he or she moves around. Veterinarians have come to use this combination therapy as one of their preferred treatments for arthritis in animals.

Cartilage from cows, pigs, chickens, or sharks is the usual source for the chondroitin supplements, while glucosamine is usually derived from crab shells. The effective dose of chondroitin is about 800 mg daily, whereas the daily dose of glucosamine is 1000 to 1500 mg daily. Look for a high-quality product that contains both substances in a single tablet. Glucosamine and chondroitin supplements are relatively expensive and have been found to be somewhat variable from product to product with respect to meeting their label claims. Go to consumerlabs.com to find an approved product.

Potassium and Magnesium

Potassium is an underappreciated antiaging supernutrient that we get too little of—just the opposite of sodium. We are designed to consume about two or three times more potassium, and only about one-sixth the sodium that we eat today. Potassium is found in high levels in vegetables, fruits, berries, nuts, soymilk, nonfat dairy, fish, and seafood. When you increase your potassium intake, you lower your blood pressure and offset the ill effects of the modern high-sodium diet. Potassium also keeps your bones strong and healthy by buffering the acid-producing effects of grains and meats. The Forever Young diet is loaded with potassium, which works wonders when combined with lean protein for making you thin and youthful again.

Magnesium is crucial for more than 300 biochemical reactions in the body and for energy production from the food we eat. Heart, nerve, muscle function, bone health, and blood clotting are also dependent upon adequate magnesium. A high magnesium intake lowers blood pressure and reduces risk of heart attack, stroke, diabetes, and osteoporosis. You need at least 400 mg daily, but many Americans do not meet this minimum requirement. To make matters worse, you absorb less magnesium as you age. So it is important to consume foods high in magnesium on a daily basis. The best sources are fish, nuts, green leafy vegetables like spinach and broccoli, seeds, beans, avocados, chocolate, soy foods, and whole grains.

In 2004, Harvard researchers published a study on 130,000 men and women that showed magnesium protected against the development of type 2 diabetes. Other studies show magnesium from dietary sources decreases risk of heart attack and stroke. The Forever Young diet is so rich in these healthy minerals it could be named the Potassium/Magnesium diet. Although potassium and magnesium are critically important nutrients, you won't need to take them in a supplement when you follow this eating style unless you are on a prescription diuretic drug.

Aspirin

> If you are feeling tense, irritable, and you
> get a headache, do what it says on the aspirin bottle:
> "Take two aspirin"
> "Keep away from children."

A highly respected expert consensus paper written by seventy doctors of the American College of Chest Physicians offers state-of-the-art advice on who should receive antiplatelet or anticoagulant drugs, commonly referred to as blood thinners. This panel of experts recommends low-dose aspirin for all people over fifty with at least one cardiovascular risk factor (male gender, high blood pressure or cholesterol, smoking, lack of exercise, family history of heart trouble, or diabetes). Aspirin clearly has been proven to be helpful in preventing against the abnormal clotting in arteries that is the usual cause of heart attack and stroke. About 100,000 men and women have been followed closely for many years after being randomly assigned in studies to aspirin or a look-alike but inactive placebo.

In composite, these studies show that aspirin will lower risk of heart attack in men by 32 percent and lower risk of stroke in women by about 19 percent. This inexpensive 100-year-old drug derived from the bark of willow trees also may protect against dementia (like Alzheimer's disease), colorectal cancer, and breast cancer. However, doses of aspirin over 81 mg daily increase the risk of ulcers and bleeding from the stomach or intestines, and also may increase risk of pancreatic cancer, an especially lethal malignancy. So we recommend that you try to limit aspirin doses to 81 mg daily, preferably not taken on an empty stomach. If you have stomach or bleeding problems or any history of aspirin-sensitivity, consult with your doctor before starting aspirin therapy. We personally take about 81 mg of aspirin every other day, which still provides cardiovascular benefits with minimal risks and side effects. Some experts believe that women do not benefit from daily low-dose aspirin unless they are over sixty-five or have other issues, such as a prior history of heart disease.

Cinnamon

Pure ground cinnamon is a spice that appears to have powerful benefits for obese people or those with elevated glucose and/or cholesterol levels who are at risk for developing diabetes. This herb, made from the dried inner bark of the shoots of a plant, has been used for over 4,000 years by populations in China, Africa, and Europe. The active ingredient in cinnamon appears to be a polyphenol (antioxidant) called MHCP, which mimics insulin and activates the insulin receptor, thereby lowering glucose in the bloodstream and improving insulin sensitivity. Adding only one-quarter to one-half of a teaspoon of cinnamon daily to the diets of people with diabetes reduced blood sugar and triglyceride levels by about 25 percent and decreased the LDL cholesterol by about 20 percent.

Cinnamon in the form of powder or capsules (but not oils) improves the body's sensitivity to insulin, which translates to better control of blood sugar and lipid levels, and it also can lower blood pressure and reduce generalized inflammation. This spice has a natural sweet flavor with no calories, and it is a great way to sweeten nonfat plain yogurt, coffee, tea, or even nonfat milk. If you don't like the taste of cinnamon, you can find capsules of it in your local health food store. You need about one gram of cinnamon daily (usually two capsules) to reap these health benefits.

The Dangers of High-Dose Vitamin E

A vitamin E supplement is not necessary since the largest and best studies show that vitamin E does not improve cardiac health. According to a large study published in the November 2004 issue of the *Annals of Internal Medicine*, high doses of vitamin E might even slightly increase risk of death. This study was a meta-analysis (a combination of all the large trials on a topic) that included over 135,000 participants in nineteen clinical trials taking doses of vitamin E ranging from 16 to 2000 IU per day. At doses of 400 IU or higher per day, a slightly increased risk (5 percent) of death was noted—with the risk increasing to 8 percent as the dose escalated up to 2000 IU. A small decrease in risk of death was noted at doses of vitamin E 100 IU or less. Like all essential nutrients, vitamin E is important for health but more is not necessarily better. When you take high doses of vitamin supplements, you often cause the levels of these substances to rise above their optimal ranges, and you may actually diminish the absorption or retention of related and potentially more beneficial nutrients from the diet.

9

GOOD THINGS FIRST: THE DIET AND LIFESTYLE FOR HEALTHY AND HAPPY KIDS

We have four kids: Jimmy, age eighteen, twelve-year-old Evan, Kathleen, age nine, and Caroline, five. With four children, three dogs, three cats, and usually a few neighbor kids bouncing around, our household is a pretty hectic place. Children know how to have fun, and we tend to feel that the more the merrier.

It is easy to recognize the blessings of this wonderful world when you can see it through the eyes of young people filled with enthusiasm, joy, and optimism. Although life always changes, we wish we could just freeze this moment in time. But we hope Caroline will always dance and Kathleen will always believe; Evan will always make sure his sisters are in a good place, Jimmy will always sing, and that we will someday have the chance to nurture our grandchildren. When we tuck the little ones into bed at night and say our prayers, we feel grateful for our family—they are the best part of who we are. That is why we take childhood nutrition so seriously. We cherish the loved ones in our lives, and do everything we can to keep them healthy and happy for the future, including making sure that the food and beverages that they consume and the lifestyle they lead will help them grow to be the best they can be.

Growing Out Before Growing Up: Childhood Obesity

Childhood obesity is increasing at an alarming rate. American children are overfed but undernourished; they consume too many empty calories but not enough beneficial nutrients. A child born in America in 2000 has a 30 to 40 percent chance of developing diabetes during his or her lifetime, largely due to excess weight, poor diet, and too little physical activity. The epidemic of obesity is even reaching down into the sandbox: more than 10 percent of children between the ages two and five are already overweight.

Fighting the battle of nutrition with your kids, as difficult as it can be, is critically important to their long-term health and happiness. If you don't do it, it won't happen. Teaching and showing them how to eat right and exercise is one of the most important gifts you can give your children. They will learn to prefer a healthy cuisine if that's what they are served regularly at home. Our Kathleen, like our other children, loves to eat fish. We have a great photo of her as a toddler in a high chair with a "cat that swallowed the canary" look on her face, smiling through pursed lips with a sardine tail poking out of her mouth. Even today, Kathleen and I will sometimes share a can of sardines for breakfast. Sure, our kids have a sweet tooth just like most children naturally do. But if you see to it that they consistently eat and drink the Forever Young way, they will lose their craving for candy and sweets by the time they get to be about five or six years old. Many parents just give up because their kids have access to junk food and candy almost everywhere they go. It's obvious you can't control what they eat when they aren't with you, but you can't use this as an excuse to abandon your responsibility to feed them healthy foods at home. What they learn to eat as their staple day-to-day diet is what they will come to prefer. If your children eat right at home and when they eat out with you, they will develop a healthy taste.

Recently Jimmy invited three of his teenage buddies over for dinner. We had a typical Forever Young meal: grilled salmon and grilled asparagus, fresh cantaloupe and strawberries, whole-grain bread with garlic oil (olive oil with fresh crushed garlic) for dipping. We drank skim or soymilk and water, and for dessert had a little dark chocolate with hot green tea. This is not what Jimmy's friends were accustomed to eating, yet they gobbled up the food just as our children do each evening. I asked the boys how they liked this style of eating, and they replied, "We love eating here, the food is awesome." Kids adapt to the Forever Young foods and beverages quickly and easily. It is the parents who often have a harder time committing to and following through with the program. The concept of what to feed your kids is pretty simple: Eat fresh, natural, whole foods as much as possible. Tell your children that they should mostly eat foods that come directly from nature. When Joan was making this point to a class of third graders, one of them asked, "Mrs. O'Keefe, can I have Bagel Bites?" She replied, "Only if they grew on a Bagel Bites tree."

They may not make the best choices at school, but you can teach your kids to develop healthy eating habits at home. After all, sixteen of the twenty-one meals they eat each week are under your control. The other day Joan was carpooling the kids and their friends home from school when Evan asked, "What's for dinner?" Joan replied, "Scallops, asparagus, tomatoes, salad, and cantaloupe for dessert." One of Kathleen's nine-year-old friends asked, "What are scallops?" "You don't know what scallops are?" exclaimed an astonished Kathleen. Children need to be repeatedly served a variety of healthful foods like seafood and vegetables in order to develop a taste for them. Natural foods are replete with great nutrients, but since each has a different nutritional profile, the best strategy is to eat a wide array of fresh whole foods.

Today, holidays and celebrations have become junk food festivals. "Don't you let your kids go trick or treating?" Joan is often asked by her clients. Of course we take the kids out on Halloween to collect candy. They come home with buckets full of sweets after they have gotten an evening's worth of great exercise and fun, running from house to house. But then there are two rules that must be followed. First, the candy is kept in a place where Mom can monitor it—like the kitchen, not their bedroom. Second, after a week at the most, the candy mysteriously disappears, usually in the trash. Use these rules not just for Halloween, but also for Valentine's Day, Easter, or any other occasion that involves candy and other sweets.

Whatever you do, don't try to get your kids on fad diets. You should *never* talk about putting your kids on a diet; this only increases the likelihood that they will binge just out of rebellion. Instead, emphasize healthy eating habits, and lead by example.

A survey conducted by the University of Minnesota asked about 4,100 middle- and high-school students what they did to drop excess pounds. More than half of the girls and one-third of the boys resorted to unhealthy tactics. The teens tried to lose weight by doing things like skipping meals, smoking, using laxatives or diuretics, and inducing vomiting. The girls especially tended to make bad food choices like skipping fruits and other whole foods.

Tell your child, "When it comes to your own body, you are the expert. Listen carefully to your body's signals of hunger and fullness. Pay attention to how you different you feel after you eat nutritious foods versus junk foods. Point out to your children that people's choices in serving sizes tend to mirror their body sizes. Joan explains to kids that when they are at the concessions counter at the movie theater and are asked, "What size popcorn do you want: small, medium, large, or tub?" that they should rephrase the question in their own mind to: "What size belly do I want?" If you can motivate them to make nutrition work for them, they will learn to make the right choices. By understanding why these steps are so important, they may come to take ownership in their own health.

Insist That the Kids Eat Breakfast

Seeing to it that your kids have a healthy breakfast every morning is one of the most important things you can do to ensure they will thrive physically and mentally. Scientific studies show that children who eat breakfast perform better in school, just as adults do better at work if they have taken time to eat a nutritious meal before starting their day. Whether you study at school, work in an office or on the farm, stay at home, or travel, it is a good idea to eat breakfast.

If your children skip the first meal of the day, they become mentally and physically tired by midmorning as their brains and bodies run low on fuel. About that time, teens will often resort to a caffeinated soda like Coke and a sugary candy bar or doughnut to wake up again. Younger kids just zone out and stop learning altogether. By lunchtime, your children are often hungry, crabby, and more prone to choose unhealthy options to eat. Starting off with a good breakfast sets the right tone for the entire day.

A healthy breakfast contains protein, fiber, phytonutrients, and water. A great way to start your child's day is a simple meal like one or two hard-boiled eggs, an orange, and a bowl of whole-grain cereal with soymilk. Stay away from the quickly digested sugary and starchy cereals, syrups, pastries, and white breads. These types of food quickly raise blood sugar (glucose) and leave kids hungry and tired one or two hours later when the glucose level comes crashing down. A breakfast high in protein, fiber, and healthy carbs (like fruit and whole grains) will smooth out blood sugar and keep your child thinking sharply until lunchtime without the distraction of hunger pangs.

If your child doesn't like to eat much for breakfast, you can split it up into two smaller meals. Serve a cup of skim milk or a glass of water with a scoop of chocolate whey protein in it while they are getting ready for school, and an orange or some berries. Don't forget a snack—an apple and two ounces of nuts—for a mid-morning break.

Active Play Is Best

A recent survey by the *Weekly Reader* asked overweight kids what triggered their overeating. Boredom, cited by 36 percent of the kids, was the number one culprit for overeating; other common triggers were stress (19 percent), watching TV (12 percent), and loneliness (9 percent). In October 2004, the Institute of Medicine called for a broad scale effort to address childhood obesity involving parents, children, schools, government, and the food and beverage industries. The institute recommended several steps likely to make a positive difference: limit time for TV and computer games to not more than two hours daily, provide healthy food at home, and set a good example for your kids.

If you are worried that your children spend too much time sitting in front of a television or computer screen, offer them a fun, active option. A recent study from Vanderbilt University found that when given the choice between an aerobic activity like swimming or soccer versus a sedentary one like watching TV or playing video games, children overwhelmingly opted for physical activity. Amazingly, even after they completed the two-month study, the more energetic lifestyle persisted. The children quickly adopted a routine of active play and preferred to stick with it rather than gravitate back to passive viewing habits. Kids naturally love to play—give them something active to do, and they will jump at the chance. Even though it might require some work on your part, try to get your children into programs involving dance, swimming, or tennis. Team sports, especially vigorous ones like soccer, basketball, and track more than baseball also offer excellent opportunities for physical activity. When developed in childhood, healthy habits like a love of physical play will hold them in good stead for their entire lives.

We make a point of going on an outing almost every day. In the summer, we walk or bike down to the local pool and go swimming to cool off in the evening. The kids love to take the puppies out for a run, or shoot baskets, or ride scooters, or sled in the winter, or ride their bikes to visit neighborhood friends or a nearby park. A recent study established that the mood-boosting effects of exercise are a key to successfully raising happy children. The researchers followed 4,500 children for two years during middle school. The kids who exercised for at least twenty minutes three or more times per week reported the lowest rates of sadness; the most sedentary children had the highest levels of despair and anxiety. Amazingly, their activity level was a stronger predictor of mood than other factors such as appearance, achievement, perceptions of health, socioeconomic status of the family, tobacco or alcohol use, or gender.

Exercise has also been shown to improve mental performance in children and adults. A study from the *Journal of Exercise Physiology* published in 2005 evaluated almost 900,000 fifth, seventh, and ninth graders and correlated their fitness level with academic performance. It found that the fittest students scored highest on the standardized achievement tests. As the fitness scores improved, the test scores improved, as well. For example, the students who were able to achieve only three of the six fitness goals scored an average math score of 48, whereas the kids who achieved all six fitness goals averaged a math score of 60. Studies show that the positive effect of aerobic exercise on learning ability occurs almost immediately. Exercise appears to change the function of the brain resulting in a short-term boost in ability to process data.

Our kids have learned that if they start acting fussy James is likely to drag them out of the house to get some activity. Jimmy will tell his brother Evan, "If you don't cheer up, Dad is going to take you out for a run." Yet no matter how cranky they are when we leave, they are always happy and relaxed by the time we come back to the house.

If you want to raise strong and confident kids, you need to pay close attention to what they are eating and how much exercise they get. A new study reported that overweight children and teens have markedly lower self-esteem than normal-weight youths. When you consider that 15 percent of American children are overweight or obese and 30 percent have the beginnings of the metabolic syndrome, this is a major issue not just for happiness but also for health. Scientists do not exactly understand why excess weight negatively impacts the self-esteem of young people, but possible factors include a less vigorous and energetic outlook, teasing from other kids or lower popularity, and disturbed hormonal levels. Help your children by encouraging them to play physically at least an hour each day. Make sure to get them involved in activities they enjoy, so they will spontaneously choose to play on their own.

It is a good idea to have your doctor track your child's weight and height on a regular basis, with measurements at least once a year that allow you to recognize and address any weight issues as soon as they develop and before they get out of hand.

> **Germs and God are everywhere.**
> **So wash your hands and say your prayers.**
> —UNKNOWN

Regular hand-washing is very important for children and adults alike. The simple act of hand-washing is the single most effective strategy for reducing the incidence of many common infectious diseases like influenza, which kills 35,000 Americans each year, and the common cold. Tell your kids to wash their hands with warm water and soap before each meal, and after each time they use the bathroom. Teach them to use a tissue and encourage them to keep their fingers away from their eyes and nose, the most common sites through which viruses enter our system and initiate infections.

Strong Bones Begin in Childhood

Bones are built when we are children. If we don't lay down strong, healthy bones as youngsters, we are destined to suffer from problems like fractures and osteoporosis as adults. A three-pronged approach is necessary to build a strong skeleton: diet, exercise, and vitamin D. You can make sure your children grow strong and sturdy bones by helping them to stay physically active. Bone cells receive the signal to grow stronger when challenged with activities such as running, climbing, jumping, and lifting. Try to get your kids to drink two glasses of nonfat milk daily and avoid soda. The phosphorus, high fructose corn syrup, and acidic nature of soda all conspire to leach the calcium out of and turn your childrens' bones to chalk. Finally, make sure they are getting enough vitamin D. Milk is fortified with this important nutrient, but about 90 percent of it is made by the skin when exposed to sunlight. So make sure they get outside to play—this will keep them happy and make their bones strong and healthy.

Omega-3: The Most Important Supplement for Kids

Omega-3 may be even more important for kids than for adults. The brain and nervous system of children are dependent upon an adequate supply of omega-3 to develop and function normally. This nutrient is so critical to the developing fetus that the body will naturally leech DHA, the most critical omega-3, from the mother's brain during pregnancy unless she is taking in sufficient quantities of this vital nutrient in her diet. Many women who do not consume adequate amounts of omega-3 while pregnant develop postpartum depression that is avoidable and reversible by taking supplements.

We give our children one daily multivitamin and two capsules of a pharmaceutical-grade omega-3 per day. Caroline, our five-year-old, can't swallow pills yet, so she gets a tablespoon of highly concentrated, lemon-flavored omega-3 about two times per week. We make sure everyone we love is getting their omega-3, even the dogs. We generally use one capsule daily of the standard inexpensive generic omega-3 for them.

Family Dining: The Gift That Keeps on Giving

The evening meal is our favorite time of the day, and we feel cheated when it doesn't happen or we miss it due to work obligations. We understand the critical importance of this family ritual, and are becoming more conscientious about making it a priority. We turn off the television, gather around the table, say a quick prayer of thanks, and share a meal. The kids tell stories, we exchange ideas and feelings, and we laugh and sometimes argue. Sure, Joan tries in vain to teach us some table manners, but mostly it is a time to relax and enjoy one anothers' company. Joan says that when you talk to your kids about the small stuff on a day-to-day basis, they will grow to trust you when they need to talk to you about the big stuff. Mealtime is a great opportunity to chat and also to help your children to appreciate their distinctive family culture and traditions.

Children subconsciously copy your behavior and generally come to share your attitudes about foods. When you cook, serve, and eat sensible portion sizes of healthy fresh foods, then they will just naturally become good eaters. These days, carving out time for family dining is not easy, but this is definitely a battle worth picking.

Unfortunately, when we get overbooked and something has to give, the family meal often is the first thing to go. For many families, this is happening more and more. Researchers from the University of Michigan Survey Research Center reported that today only one out of every three American families dines together in the evening, compared to about two out of three families thirty years ago. The average duration of these mealtimes is also dwindling, down about 10 percent since 1981. This is a worrisome trend because family mealtime somehow represents something much more than just a few moments to share food. Research shows that dining together as a family is an important step toward ensuring good physical and mental health for your children.

The scientific research on the importance of family meals is nothing short of astounding. A widely quoted *Reader's Digest* national poll dating back to 1994 showed that high-school seniors who achieved higher scholastic scores tended to dine with their families more frequently as they were growing up. A more recent University of Michigan study confirmed this finding and showed that the amount of time children spent eating with their families was the *single most powerful predictor* of higher standardized test scores and lower likelihood of behavior difficulties. Amazingly, regular family dining predicted student test scores more accurately than time devoted to studying, attending classes, going to religious services, or participating in athletic, musical, or artistic activities.

It is also becoming clear that kids who eat meals at home tend to consume a more nutritious diet. A Harvard study in the March 2000 *Archives of Family Medicine* found that frequent family dining was associated with a healthier diet. Specifically, the families who ate together on all or most days of the week typically consumed higher quantities of essential nutrients like fiber, calcium, iron, vitamins, and minerals and also ate less unhealthy fat compared to families who never or rarely ate together. Other studies show that children who eat family meals consume more vegetables and fruits and fewer snack foods than kids who did not share meals with their families.

University of Minnesota researchers reported in the *Archives of Pediatrics and Adolescent Medicine* in August 2004 that frequent family dining also reduced the likelihood of drug and alcohol abuse and unhealthy weight-control practices in young people. Another survey of high-achieving teens found that those who ate meals with their family on a regular basis tended to be happier with their present life and their prospects for the future. The benefits of family dining are apparent regardless of the time of day the meals occurred. If you are having a hard time getting everyone together for dinner, perhaps you should try to start the tradition of a family breakfast each morning.

Activities Displace Family Time

In an excellent article that appeared in the January 4, 2005, issue of *USA Today*, William Mattox Jr. discussed how parenting has become like a competitive sport with trophies awarded to the busiest. He wrote, "Parents today have so many extracurricular activities that there's little room for such family activities as dinners, vacations, weekend outings, and visits to relatives. And this wouldn't be so worrisome if the family activities weren't so important to the well-being of the children." The main culprit that is disrupting family mealtime is no mystery to anyone who is raising kids today. After-school activities have both parents and children running around like chickens with their heads cut off. William Doherty wrote an essay on this topic in the book *Take Back Your Time*. He reported that children today are spending more than twice as much time each week playing organized sports as they did in 1981. However, the amount of time they spend passively watching siblings' activities (like brother's baseball game or sister's piano recital) has increased sixfold over the same time frame.

A survey from the Surface Transportation Policy Project of 2004 found that the average mom now spends more time driving each day than eating with her family. When we trade in our family meals for fast food, we lose the vegetables and fruits and gain weight. And it is not just the nutrition that suffers; the entire family dynamic is compromised, and for what?

It may be true that if you want your son to be the next Tiger Woods, he will have to play golf for hours every day from the time he can walk. But he will only be a kid once, and spending his childhood in an apprenticeship for adulthood is not the recipe for a well-adjusted and happy person. We have no illusions about our children someday making a living in professional sports. The odds against making the big leagues are minuscule even for athletically gifted children. Yet parents often end up sacrificing perhaps their most sacred family bonding time to these trivial activities.

Joan's policy is only one sport per season, and if the child doesn't really love a particular activity—it's gone. It's true that sports activities are usually great for exercise, and we try to steer our kids into those that involve continual motion—like basketball, swimming, running, and soccer—that tend to expend a lot of energy. We try to avoid traveling teams—until the kids get into high school—and activities that require excessive time commitments, especially around supper time.

Unstructured playtime is not only more fun for the kids, it is better for fostering creativity in their developing minds. Many parents are increasingly nervous about the safety of their children while playing in the neighborhood. This is a usually a misperception fueled by the hype-hungry media that tell us about the horrible crimes against children that are usually irrelevant to your neighborhood. Statistically speaking, there has never been a safer time for a child to be alive than today. Playing outside with siblings or friends or parents is one of the best things a kid can do. Put a basketball hoop up in your driveway and make your own yard a playground.

Your Children Are Watching You Closely

They consciously and subconsciously pattern their lives after yours: how you eat, what you do in your free time, your attitude about life, how you treat other people. Kids tend to do what you do, not what you say. If you want active, healthy, and fit children, you need to walk the walk, or run the run, or swim the swim, and not just talk the talk. If you can't motivate yourself to exercise, maybe the knowledge that your child's health is at stake will inspire you to get off the couch and get moving. A new study tracked 150 children from birth to explore the critical factors in determining excess weight gain. Over two out of three of the kids who became overweight had parents who were also overweight; only 16 percent of children with two normal-weight parents developed a weight problem. While some of this tendency to develop obesity is genetic, the researchers found that more of it was related to lifestyle issues like a diet of high-calorie foods and beverages and not enough physical activity.

Help for Your Teen's Complexion Problems

Dr. Loren Cordain has done pioneering work to show that a hunter-gatherer diet, such as the Forever Young program, will even clear up almost any complexion suprisingly well—despite decades of dermatologists' advice telling us that acne, the scourge of the modern teenager, has nothing to do with diet. It all depends on what diet you use. If it is the diet that we are designed to thrive upon, it will make your adolescent's skin clear and healthy again without having to resort to potentially dangerous prescription medications like antibiotics and Accutane. Get your kids to eat the Forever Young way and they will have beautiful skin.

> **Tip:** *Try to keep healthy snacks around the house to offer the kids when they get hungry. Apples, carrots, oranges, tangerines, nectarines, berries, string cheese, milk, and nuts all make delicious snacks that most children just naturally love. It may take some time to wean them from the junk food, but you will find it easier to get them hooked on good foods if they aren't tempted by the cookies, candy, and chips in the cupboards and Coke in the refrigerator.*

Turn Off the TV and Tune In to a Healthier Life

The latest surveys show that children now watch about three hours of television per day. Over the course of one year, the average American child spends more time watching television than in school. In fact, next to sleeping, kids spend more time watching TV than any other single activity. Too much television has been linked to poor school performance, sleep and behavior problems, and obesity. Believe it or not, the basal metabolic rate (how many calories your child is burning at rest) is lower while viewing TV than when sleeping. To make matters worse, the ads are often promoting unhealthy, high-calorie foods like candy and soda. A Harvard study published in *Pediatrics* in December 2003 found that the more TV a child watched the fewer fruits and vegetables he or she consumed on a daily basis. Research consistently shows that kids who spend more than ten hours weekly watching TV are most likely to be overweight.

A child's room is no place for a television or a computer with Internet access. A study published in the June 2002 issue of the journal *Pediatrics* showed that children ages one to five with a television in their room watched TV five hours more per week than kids without a TV in their room. This study of more than 2,700 children also found that the likelihood of obesity was one-third higher in the children who had a TV in their room. The National Institute of Child Health and Human Development conducted a survey of twelve- to sixteen-year-olds and found that kids with a television in their room were two times more likely to smoke marijuana, one-third more likely to drink alcohol, and 50 percent more likely to be sexually active than those without one.

TV viewing usually displaces other activities that are generally more fun and productive, like spending time with family and friends, playing actively, getting fresh air, reading, doing homework, and finishing chores. Childhood is a unique phase of our lives during which our brains are particularly capable of soaking up knowledge and developing new skills. Youngsters have capacities for mastering disciplines such as music, language, sports, art, and even play. If these aptitudes are not tapped in childhood, they probably will never fully develop in adulthood. It seems such a shame to waste these precious, irreplaceable years by just passively vegging out in front of a screen instead of nurturing a child's true potential.

The American Academy of Pediatrics recommends that children's viewing time be limited to one or two hours per day. Or some parents may limit TV to one hour on school nights and two or three hours on weekends. Make specific rules about when and where your children can watch TV; for example, no TV during meals, homework, or when friends come over to play. Television viewing habits are another issue that is taught best by example. Turn off the TV and find some fun, stimulating things you and your kids can do together.

10

PRESCRIPTION DRUGS THAT IMPROVE LONGEVITY

Most people underestimate the power they have to control their health and longevity. At least 70 percent of aging and disease is a function of lifestyle (diet and exercise) and attitude. A landmark study published in September 2004 in *The Lancet* evaluated 30,000 people from fifty-two different countries to firmly establish the factors that account for the growing worldwide epidemic of heart disease. The authors found that nine risk factors, all of them modifiable, accounted for 94 percent of heart attacks in women and 90 percent in men. The factors that were responsible for nearly all of the heart attacks included high cholesterol, smoking, high blood pressure, diabetes, obesity (especially in and around the abdomen), emotional stress, a diet low in vegetables and fruit, abstinence from alcohol use, and lack of exercise. Some of these are just a matter of prioritizing lifestyle decisions, but others, like cholesterol levels and blood pressure, often require medications. The bottom line is very good news: If you pay attention to these risk factors, you can almost guarantee that heart disease, the number one cause of death and disability in our society, will not get you.

We tell people who have naturally low blood pressure and great cholesterol levels that they should take good care of themselves because they are going to be around for a long time. But even if you don't have ideal genes, there are medications that can safely get your numbers into the ranges that will keep your heart, blood vessels, and brain vigorous and youthful even into your eighties and nineties.

Blood Pressure Meds and Statins: Correction Factors for Stresses of the Modern World

Statistically, about 50 percent of us (both men and women) are destined to die from cardiovascular illness, which are almost entirely preventable. All the steps in the Forever Young program that will keep your weight down and your heart healthy also appear to help prevent the other diseases of aging like high blood pressure, Alzheimer's, osteoporosis, and cancer.

If you do have abnormal lipids or high blood pressure you have plenty of company—it's almost the norm in our society today. About nine out of ten Americans develop high blood pressure sooner or later. The average cholesterol in American adults is 208 mg/dL, or about twice the truly normal level. If your cholesterol and/or blood pressure are too high, don't be like an ostrich and take a head-in-the-sand approach. When you ignore these silent killers, mope about your bad luck, and quit taking your blood pressure and cholesterol pills, you are only cheating yourself out of a long and healthy life. If your diet and lifestyle changes aren't enough, there are safe and effective medications to bring these numbers into their ideal ranges.

Our patients often tell us, "I don't want to be dependent on drugs. They might poison my body." We firmly believe that natural is best when it comes to treating any health problem. The exercise and diet program, weight loss, stress reduction, and smoking cessation strategies outlined in this book are all great for improving risk factors. Unfortunately, these natural therapies, important as they are, often aren't enough to normalize high blood pressure or abnormal cholesterol levels.

If you had life-threatening pneumonia or some other serious bacterial infection, I suspect you wouldn't refuse to take an antibiotic. The "miracle drugs" of the twenty-first century—statins to lower cholesterol, and modern blood pressure medications—have power to keep your arteries soft, smooth, and youthful rather than inflamed, hardened, and clogged. Since these pills can undo much of the damage inherent in our contemporary lifestyle, by forgoing them, you deprive yourself of one the unique advantages of living in the modern world.

"Lower is better" is the mantra of enlightened physicians and medical scientists today. The ability to safely and effectively keep your numbers down, way down, is emerging as one of the most powerful antiaging strategies. Specifically, we are talking about achieving and maintaining optimal levels of cholesterol, blood pressure, weight, daily calorie intake, and blood glucose. Only recently—thanks to remarkable scientific advances in the pharmaceutical industry—has this become a possibility for virtually everyone. The diet and exercise sections of the Forever Young program will help you achieve your ideal weight, calorie intake, and blood glucose targets.

It may seem a little radical to suggest that you take prescription drugs to delay the ravages of age on your heart, brain, and arteries, but this is the one of the most important steps you can take to ensure a long and healthy life. The optimal range for both the systolic (top) blood pressure and total cholesterol level is about 95 to 125. These were the normal levels in humans when we were living in our indigenous hunter-gatherer world. Recent scientific studies demonstrate clearly that when we keep blood pressure and cholesterol below 120, we prevent the scourges of modern civilization—premature disease and aging of the blood vessels, heart, and brain. Most adult Americans have cholesterol and blood pressure levels above the optimal ranges. As the years pass, these stresses cause the arteries and heart to thicken and stiffen, hallmarks of an old cardiovascular system. Although this occurs at different rates in all of us, most people will sooner or later develop hardening of the arteries. Fortunately, we have a statin for your cholesterol and medications for your blood pressure to prevent much aging of the cardiovascular system and brain. The standard approach is to reserve these miracle drugs for those who suffer cardiovascular events like heart attack or stroke, or those with very elevated blood and cholesterol levels. Instead, we are suggesting that you proactively normalize these important parameters to prevent disease and aging before severe disabilities occur.

Thus, we like to think of statins and modern blood pressure drugs as "correction factors" for living in the modern world. With the help of one or more of these medications, most people can achieve longevity with vigor and avoid most of the common diseases of aging such as heart attack, stroke, Alzheimer's disease, osteoporosis, and macular degeneration, regardless of their genetic makeup.

Blood Pressure Meds

Even if you aren't one of the lucky few blessed with lifelong low blood pressure, you can keep your arteries, heart, kidneys, and brain youthful by taking one or more of the safe and effective blood pressure–lowering drugs. Our favorites are the ACEs (angiotensin converting enzyme inhibitors) and the ARBs (angiotensin receptor blockers). These drugs are well tolerated and have been extensively studied. When physicians need a blood pressure drug personally, they usually choose to take an ACE or an ARB because these medications work well and are relatively easy to tolerate. The ARBs are expecially well tolerated with no more side effects than a placebo. By reversing the overgrowth of fibrous muscle tissue in the heart and blood vessels that occurs with age, ACEs and ARBs prevent hardening of the arteries. However, recent studies have concluded that the most important thing about blood pressure is getting it down—not which medication you are taking to accomplish this goal.

John is a patient and friend who at age forty-eight began to notice fatigue, headaches, and skipped heartbeats. His blood pressure had always been very normal at about 115/70, but now it was running in the high normal range (about 130 to 139 over 80). After taking an ARB, his blood pressure is now 114/68. His energy level quickly returned to normal, and now he virtually never has headaches or palpitations from irregular heartbeats. ACE inhibitors and ARBs reduce the occurrences of many common medical problems—strokes, congestive heart failure, heart attacks, headaches (particularly migraines), atrial fibrillation (a rapid, chaotic, heart rhythm that predisposes to stroke and heart failure), kidney disease, and dementia. Atrial fibrillation in particular is an increasingly common problem. A study published in August 2004 in *Circulation* found that about 25 percent of Americans will develop atrial fibrillation during their lifetime. ACEs and ARBs help to prevent this dangerous rhythm, in part by keeping the blood vessels and heart soft and supple—as they are in healthy teenagers. This makes your heart and arteries flexible and less irritable, which reduces rhythm problems and headaches.

Surprisingly, ACEs and ARBs also decrease your risk of developing type 2 diabetes, one of the most dangerous and prevalent health problems today, by about 25 percent to 30 percent. We are still uncertain how ACEs and ARBs prevent diabetes, but this phenomenon has been noted consistently in many large randomized trials. If you are overweight or obese, have a family history of diabetes, or have high triglycerides and low HDL cholesterol, you should probably be on an ARB or an ACE, especially if your systolic blood pressure (the top number) is over 130.

If your systolic blood pressure stays above 130 on an ARB or an ACE we often add a low dose of a mild diuretic (fluid pill) like hydrochlorothiazide (HCTZ) to bring the blood pressure down to ideal levels.

Beta-blockers (like Toprol-XL, Zebeta, Coreg, Lopressor, atenolol, and others) are another life-saving class of blood pressure drugs. By blocking the actions of adrenaline, beta-blockers lower the heart rate and blood pressure. They also reduce the risk of heart attack, congestive heart failure, and sudden death from dangerous heart rhythms. These drugs are especially important if you've had a heart attack, a history of weak heart muscle (cardiomyopathy), or congestive heart failure. In people with these problems, beta-blockers have been shown to dramatically improve longevity. Among the beta-blocker class of medications, Coreg (carvedilol) has shown the most impressive results for improving survival and overall cardiovascular health. Some of the exhilaration of life is mediated through adrenaline and other catecholamines. Consequently, when we block the effects of adrenaline by using beta-blockers, many people complain of fatigue and lethargy, loss of interest in sex, and mild depression. For this reason, beta-blockers are not agents we recommend as first-line therapy for high blood pressure. Amlodipine (Norvasc) and other calcium channel blockers are safe and effective for lowering blood pressure, especially in combination with an ACE or an ARB.

When Average Is Not Optimal

One of my favorite mentors during cardiology training used to tell me that cholesterol was overrated and essentially useless as a risk factor because almost everyone he saw with coronary artery disease had "normal" cholesterol levels. What he didn't appreciate was that virtually no one he saw had a truly normal cholesterol level. The ideal LDL cholesterol level is in the range of 50 to 70. This is what your LDL was when you were born. Currently, only about 2 percent of adult men and 5 percent of adult women have LDL cholesterol levels below 70; and the average LDL is about 135, which is approximately twice the optimal level. Coronary disease in our population remains an epidemic; about 40 percent of us still die from it. In contrast, an LDL level above 70 is uncommon among animals and humans living in their natural environment, and so is atherosclerosis—the disease of the arteries that kills so many of us today.

Statins: The Antiaging Miracle Drug

If you are a typical American your total cholesterol is about 200, which is the average level. However, when it comes to cholesterol, average is not normal. The truly normal human cholesterol is 100 to 140. For thousands of generations, our ancient ancestors lived their entire lives with cholesterol levels in this range. Among the rare tribes of humans who were still living this lifestyle up until fifty years ago, the average cholesterol value was 124. Your cholesterol was about 70 to 100 when you were born, and it started to rise as you were weaned from your mother's milk and began to eat the unnatural diet that has become the standard in our culture. The fact that your cholesterol level of 200 is average when everyone around you also has a cholesterol level that is twice the truly normal number is of no consolation to your arteries, heart, and brain. With modern imaging technology like MRI and high-speed CT scanners, most of us have arteries that are thickened with plaque by the time we are forty or fifty. Atherosclerosis is the silent stalker. In two out of three people, the first recognizable symptom of this disease is a catastrophe like heart attack, stroke, or even sudden death. That's why we often recommend that people get a Cardioscan (fast CT scan) to discover plaques and halt their progressioin long before they can cause trouble.

Our strongest weapons against the deadly atherosclerosis are the statins, an amazing class of drugs that include agents such as atorvastatin (Lipitor), simvastatin (Zocor), and rosuvastatin (Crestor). There are more randomized placebo-controlled trials testing statins that any other drug in history, and these trials have proven them to be very effective at lowering cholesterol. The studies also show that statins are very safe and well-tolerated drugs and will not "rot" your liver or cause cancer or arthritis. Statins are available over the counter in England now, and may some-day be available over the counter in the United States as well. In fact, statins are safer than many over-the-counter medications like aspirin or acetaminophen. Occasionally people on statins have trouble with muscle aches, but randomized tri-als of tens of thousands of patients show that a similar number of those receiving a placebo also complain of muscle aches. The major side effect of statins is rhab-domyolysis, or serious muscle damage, which occurs at a rate of less than one per 20,000, and is fatal in about one in 10 million. Coenzyme Q10 is an antioxidant that is naturally produced by the body. Some evidence suggests that taking a sup-plement of coenzyme Q10 might improve statin-related muscle aches. A small study presented at the March 2005 American College of Cardiology meeting showed that 85 percent of people who were complaining of muscle pain on a statin improved when they were given 100 mg of coenzyme Q10 daily.

Sales of the number-one selling statin Lipitor are $12 billion yearly, about twice as much as the second-place drug, and more than the Gross Domestic Product for many third-world nations. Cardiologists prescribe Lipitor and other statins fre-quently, and many of us now take a statin ourselves. Our cardiology journals are full of articles about the ever-expanding benefits of these miracle drugs. We see firsthand how safe and effective they are, not just for preventing heart disease but for possibly preventing many other common serious problems as well. If your cho-lesterol level is not optimal, you should take a statin and embrace this opportunity to prevent arterial aging and improve your health and longevity.

When the bad cholesterol drops below 70, the inflamed and dangerous lesions in your arteries begin to melt away. Heart attacks, strokes, and deaths from coro-nary disease dramatically decrease when we achieve and maintain LDL cholesterol of 40 to 70, which corresponds to total cholesterol of about 100 to 140. The stronger statins reduce cholesterol and inflammation, and Lipitor is the most pop-ular, Vytorin, Zocor, and Crestor are other very effective and potent statins.

Statins may also help to prevent many of the other diseases commonly attributed to the normal aging process such as macular degeneration (the most common cause of blindness), cataracts, glaucoma, some forms of dementia, multiple sclerosis, kidney failure, and maybe even osteoporosis and bone fractures. These drugs improve the function of the blood vessels and keep your arteries soft and supple. By maintaining the health of blood vessels throughout the body, statin therapy has also been shown to decrease the risk of developing erectile dysfunction.

Two studies published in the *New England Journal of Medicine* in January 2005 found that inflammation may be just as important as cholesterol in causing heart attacks and strokes. The statins not only lower cholesterol but also reduce inflammation. This one-two punch may account for the statins' remarkable abilities in improving long-term health.

The scientific community likes to theorize about special properties of statins that explain their wide variety of benefits, many of which appear unrelated to improvement in artery health. Diseases that have previously been attributed to aging may in part be a consequence of decades of living with a cholesterol twice the truly normal level. Statins bring your cholesterol back toward the physiologically normal range, which provides healing and antiaging effects that resonate throughout your system—helping to keep you young, vigorous, and mentally sharp. So, if you have a cholesterol issue, get over any phobias you might have about taking a statin; they are one of our most potent antiaging medications. In the future we will be using statins routinely as preventative medicine for people over forty-five or fifty. If you have cardiac risk factors or other issues that increase your chances of heart trouble, ask your doctor about a statin.

Rimonabant (Accomplia): A Magic Bullet for Weight Loss?

Weight loss with diet alone is a difficult proposition for many individuals. Even with popular structured programs, most people struggle to lose weight and keep it off. In a study published in the *Journal of the American Medical Association* in January 2005, the average person following Weight Watchers, the Zone diet, the Atkins diet, or the Ornish diet diligently for one year lost only five or six pounds. The weight-loss drugs that have been available to date have not been very effective in the long term either. In 2001, Keith Haddock, PhD, a friend and colleague at the Mid America Heart Institute, published a meta-analysis of the entire scientific literature on trials using weight-loss drugs. This analysis found that in over 100 randomized controlled trials, not a single drug showed a lasting weight loss over nine pounds. Although many of these compounds promise a quick and easy cure for excess weight, most of them are ineffective and potentially dangerous.

Recently, doctors in preventive cardiology and nutrition have become hopeful about rimonabant (Accomplia), a drug that is under development but not yet on the market. Rimonabant, potentially the most promising weight-loss drug ever, represents a new class of medications with a completely novel mechanism of action that blocks the cannabinoid (CB1) receptors in the brain. These receptors, which are part of the endocannabinoid system, when stimulated by marijuana, cause an altered state of consciousness and trigger cravings for food and cigarettes. Obese individuals tend to have more cannabinoid receptors than thin people. Studies with rimonabant (nicknamed the "Munchies Drug") indicate that blocking these receptors reduces cravings for junk food and cigarettes. People taking the drug reported that they felt less hungry, which led to a reduction in calorie intake, thereby enhancing weight loss.

At the November 2004 American Heart Association meeting, results of the North American trial of rimonabant were presented. The study was a placebo-controlled trial evaluating the effects of rimonabant on obese patients. At the end of two years, the people receiving the 20 mg dose lost an average of 8.7 kilograms (19 pounds) and 3.4 inches off their waist measurement.

Rimonabant may be the first practical and effective weight-loss drug. We are coming to view obesity as a chronic relapsing medical condition, similar to high blood pressure, high cholesterol, or diabetes. As with most chronic diseases, long-term control of obesity will likely need long-term treatment, and rimonabant will probably be continued chronically to keep the excess weight from reaccumulating. More studies are under way, but this is definitely an agent with tremendous potential. Not only because it may make you look and feel better, but also because it helps to reverse two of the most serious health issues today—abdominal obesity and the metabolic syndrome (insulin resistance). Rimonabant appears to be the most effective drug therapy yet for improving obesity and its related metabolic disorders. It also helps people quit smoking, while at the same time blunting the customary weight gain noted upon tobacco withdrawal.

The Dark Side of Rimonabant

Both the medical profession and the general public have been keenly interested in the developing story of rimonabant. If this drug is approved by the FDA, it will likely be a blockbuster generating millions of prescriptions in a short time. One of James's mentors at the Mayo Clinic used to jokingly tell us that he used new drugs for only the first year or two after they were released—before they had the chance to develop any serious side effects. Although rimonabant seems to be reasonably safe now, we often cannot fully appreciate the safety profile of a drug until large numbers of people have been on it for a few years.

There are two potential reasons why rimonabant should be closely scrutinized for safety issues. First, it is the first of a brand-new class of drugs that works by temporarily altering function of the endocannabinoid system, which is involved with pleasure, pain tolerance, relaxation, and oral cravings. So far, rimonabant appears to reduce the munchies and cravings for nicotine, while causing relatively few serious side effects, although depression has been reported in a small percentage of people on the drug. Second, a few worrisome reactions have occurred among the thousands of subjects who have taken this drug in prerelease studies. Two people have reported reversible amnesia (memory loss) while on rimonabant that resolved when the drug was stopped. Some neurologists worry that blocking the endocannabinoid system might leave the brain more susceptible to damage under the stress of stroke, traumatic brain injury, or other chronic neurological diseases. Indeed, one person with multiple sclerosis developed worsening neurological symptoms while on rimonabant. So we would urge caution about embracing this potentially exciting new agent too quickly.

Other weight-loss drugs including Xenical and Meridia are only modestly effective, have frequent and troublesome side effects, and are expensive. For the most part, we do not use these agents for our patients and do not recommend them for you.

The Dangers of Stimulant Weight-Loss Supplements

You can lose weight by a variety of means. The program described in this book will not just make you lean again, it will also make you healthier, stronger, and in many ways younger. Many other weight-loss methods will leave you lighter, but not necessarily healthier. Take up smoking, and you will lose weight. A serious cocaine or methamphetamine habit will burn up any excess fat on your body as you struggle with a potentially lethal addiction.

James first met Samantha when she was a perky, beautiful fifteen-year-old who had just recently received a heart transplant. Her own heart failed inexplicably, and she nearly died before we found a healthy replacement. Samantha did well over the ensuing six years, though she was a free spirit with a strong will who could sometimes be a bit of a rebel. She grew into a delightful young woman who was attending college in the hope of eventually going to medical school.

Suddenly, without warning, one June morning Samantha came to the emergency department of our Mid America Heart Institute at Saint Luke's Hospital with florid heart failure again. We were perplexed because she had been doing so well and was completely free of serious post-transplantation problems like organ rejection (by the patient's own immune system) or blockage of her coronary arteries. But now, she had a blood pressure of 85/50 and her heart was racing along at 115 beats per minute as she gasped for every breath. The echocardiogram showed her heart pump to be severely weakened, but the biopsy of her heart showed no signs of rejection. James frantically tried to resolve this dilemma and halt her downward spiral, but Samantha continued to deteriorate during those first few hours after her admission.

We had to be missing something—the puzzle seemed to lack a crucial piece. James sat at her bedside as she struggled to breathe. "Samantha, have you been taking any street drugs, cocaine, methamphetamines, Ectasy?" he asked. She shook her head. "How about over-the-counter weight-loss supplements like Metabolife, ephedra, or ma huang?" he queried. "Well, I have been taking ephedrine to lose about ten pounds for swimsuit season," she replied. "How much and for how long?" I asked. "About two tablets twice a day for the last five or six weeks." I pushed her for more information. "Is this the first time you have taken ephedrine?" "No," she said, "I also used it once before when I was fifteen, for a couple of months before I needed my heart transplant."

The red flags and flashing lights went off in James's mind. She had trashed her transplanted heart now, as she had her native heart six years ago, by using a powerful over-the-counter amphetamine-like substance in an effort to take off a few extra pounds. She had never confided this to us previously, and unfortunately it was too late for Samantha by this time. Despite our best efforts, we could not find another heart in time, nor could we turn her course around with drugs. She died that day at age twenty-one.

Ephedra and ephedrine were initially taken off the market in 2004 because of cardiovascular complications like those Samantha suffered. James has seen about twelve patients who have experienced life-threatening reactions to ephedrine, including a thirty-two-year-old father who was using a body-building supplement and died suddenly as a result of a lethal rhythm-ventricular tachycardia.

Ephedrine is now available again in smaller doses, and many other dangerous stimulants like synephrine, bitter orange, and pseudoephedrine, marketed for weight loss, are also available over the counter. You should avoid any temptation to try these "easy and effective" solutions to your weight problem. They are dangerous and not a long-term solution. Like cocaine or amphetamines, these compounds powerfully stimulate your heart, raise blood pressure and heart rate, and predispose you to weakened heart muscle and lethal cardiac rhythm problems. The Forever Young diet and exercise plan will help you lose weight and keep it off without resorting to the use of dangerous chemicals.

Drugs That Can Increase Weight

Some prescription drugs can increase the likelihood that you will gain weight. This table is a guide that outlines the major potential problem medications that can produce weight gain. If you are taking any of these drugs and are having weight problems, talk to your doctor about managing them.

Medication	Chance of Weight Gain		
	1-3%	4-10%	>10%
Antidepressants			
Tricyclic antidepressants such as amitriptyline (*Elavil*), desipramine (*Norpramine*), imipramine (*Norfranil*)			X
Selective serotonin-reuptake inhibitors (SSRIs) such as fluoxetine (*Prozac*), paroxetine (*Paxil*), sertraline (*Zoloft*)		X	

Medication	Chance of Weight Gain		
	1-3%	4-10%	>10%
Antidiabetic Drugs			
Insulin; sulfonylureas such as chlorpropamide (*Diabinese*), glipizide (*Glucotrol*), glyburide (*Micronase*)			X
TZDs such as pioglitazone (*Actos*) or rosiglitazone (*Avandia*)			X
Anticonvulsant Drugs			
Divalproex (*Depakote*); gabapentin (*Neurotin*)		X	
Oxcarbazepin (*Trileptal*)	X		
Antihistamine			
Azelastine nasal spray (*Astelin*)	X		
Anti-Inflammatory Drugs			
Corticosteroids such as cortisone (*Cortone*), hydrocortisone (*Cortef*), prednisone (*Deltasone*)			X
Asthma Drugs			
Inhaled corticosteroids: beclomethasone (*Vanceril*), budesonide (*Pulmicort*), flunisolide (*Aerobid*), triamcinolone (*Azmacort*)	X		
Osteoporosis Drugs			
Raloxifene (*Evista*)		X	

Medication	Chance of Weight Gain		
	1-3%	4-10%	>10%
Psychiatric Drugs			
Clozapine (*Clozaril*), olanzapine (*Zyprexa*), (*Geodon, Abilify*)			X
Quetiapine (*Seroquel*), riseperiodone (*Risperdal*)	X		
Other: Mirtazapine (*Remeron*)		X	

Source: *Consumer Reports on Health,* June 2004

PART II

The Forever Young Lifestyle

11

BECOMING HEALTHY
AND ATTRACTIVE
FROM THE INSIDE OUT

Both women and men today spend a great deal of time and money trying to recapture the healthy glow and vigor of youth. However, these fall into the category of "things that money can't buy." Whether it's a clear and radiant complexion, a strong and confident posture, an attractive smile, or a sparkle in your eyes, the right diet and lifestyle is the surest way to become more attractive.

The American Waist-land

Most Americans struggle with weight gain especially around the midsection, accumulating belly and back fat. These are the most dangerous spots to pack on fat and the most unbecoming. A narrow waist in females and a flat and muscled abdomen in males have been standards for beauty and attractiveness down through the ages, just as they are today. We have always instinctively known what science has only recently discovered: Belly fat is a sign of a disturbed metabolic/hormonal profile, the presence of excess stress hormones like insulin and cortisol, and not enough of the normal youthful sex hormones. Lean muscular men and narrow-waisted women are sexy because they have the body shape that signals a youthful and healthy constitution.

The best way to regain your youthful shape and attractiveness is from the inside out. When you follow the Forever Young program, the fat around your trunk will melt away and your bones and muscles will grow stronger. Your eyes will be brighter, and your teeth and gums will be healthier. You will become more attractive because your system is becoming healthy again as your stress hormones and free radicals plummet, and your youth-enhancing hormones and age-defying antioxidants rise. There is no shortcut to recovering the look and the glow of youth, so you will have to invest some time and energy, but the payoff is worth the effort.

A Clear and Radiant Complexion

The personal characteristics considered most attractive like a clear and smooth complexion, a clean healthy smile, full shiny hair, a toned and lean body, good posture, and bright eyes are also indicators of a strong, healthy constitution. It is easy to have these features when you are an active seventeen-year-old. After twenty-one, there really is only one way to attain this look—you have to earn it with the right diet, exercise, and lifestyle.

Don't you know someone with that vibrant, clear, beautiful skin? This asset is not a coincidence but the reflection of a hormonally balanced system that imparts a beauty and youthful glow from the inside out. You can spend all of your free time applying makeup, getting facials at the spa, and even investing in cosmetic surgery, but these will not result in the glow that comes from following the Forever Young program. When you go with the flow of the typical American lifestyle, eating too many calories, too much sugar and starch, not enough antioxidants, fiber, and fluid, you are destined to have a gray, dull, bumpy, doughy complexion that prematurely ages you.

Oral Hygiene: Crucial for Both Health and Appearance

Your teeth and gums speak volumes about your overall health, and a beautiful smile is important for appearance and comfort. Chronic infections like cavities and gingivitis and more serious periodontal diseases are closely related to serious health issues like heart disease and diabetes. In a twelve-year study of over 14,000 men, Harvard researchers found that those with the healthiest teeth and gums were the least likely to suffer a heart attack or stroke. To keep both your smile and your body healthy, floss once or twice daily and brush your teeth at least two times daily. Also consider using antibiotic toothpaste such as Colgate Total.

Most of the deeply pigmented, plant-based antiaging antioxidants like those found in purple grapes and red wine, berries, dark chocolate, tea, and coffee are among the worst culprits for superficially staining your teeth. If this becomes an issue for you, we recommend that you use nonabrasive whitening toothpaste to keep your smile bright. However, we are concerned about chronic use of bleaching systems. The active ingredient in most whitening gels is carbamide peroxide—a harsh bleaching compound that produces dangerous oxygen-free radicals that could possibly increase risk of oral cancer. On the other hand, whitening toothpastes appear to be safe. An attractive smile radiates an aura of vibrant health, just as surely as poor dental and gum health sends an unmistakable message of being unwell.

The metabolic syndrome (waist over thirty-five inches for women, forty inches for men; blood pressure over 130/85; high triglycerides, low HDL cholesterol; fasting blood sugar over 100) and diabetes frequently cause inflammation and infection of the gums. In fact, the dentist or periodontist is frequently the first one to uncover previously unrecognized diabetes or prediabetes in their patients.

In a study reported in *Circulation* dated March 9, 2004, researchers found that oral infections like cavities, gingivitis, and periodontal disease were more powerful predictors of who would develop coronary heart disease than traditional risk factors like cholesterol. Studies also show a sevenfold increase in premature delivery in pregnant women who have gum disease. Poor dental health correlates with osteoporosis, a very common problem in women past menopause. The infections in the mouth cause inflammation that can wreak havoc throughout your system. It is not known whether the bacteria themselves migrate from the mouth through the bloodstream to affect organs like the bones, heart, and uterus, or whether the inflammation itself gives off detrimental cytokines (chemical messengers) that cause the problems.

The important point is that keeping your mouth healthy will pay off big dividends in your overall health. This works both ways: If you eat the right diet, stay fit, and follow the Forever Young program, you will notice big improvements in your dental health.

The Eyes: A Window to Your Health

Healthy vision is not to be taken for granted. The eyes have been called the window to your soul, but they also provide telling insights about your physical health. Cataracts, macular degeneration, and glaucoma are very common problems in Americans as they age. The Forever Young program will help keep your eyes healthy. The hormones and pro-oxidant free radicals that rise as you become chronically overweight and overstressed "cook" the proteins in your eyes (analogous to the clouding that occurs as you heat an egg white) and can damage and destroy your eyesight. Recently, studies indicate that eye problems including cataracts and age-related macular degeneration are associated with a shortened life expectancy. By reducing calorie intake and increasing your antioxidant defenses with at least nine servings of fruits and vegetables daily, you will prevent the cooking of the proteins in your eyes and throughout your system—proteins that are vital for sharp vision and optimal longevity. Statins have been associated with decreased risk of developing macular degeneration, cataracts, and even glaucoma. You should wear sunglasses routinely when you are outside—the darker they are and the more they cover your entire field of vision, the better.

Stand Up Straight, Shoulders Back, Suck in That Gut

Carry yourself with a straight, strong posture and you will convey a youthful, confident aura. On the other hand, a stooped, round-shouldered slouch adds decades to your perceived age. The pull of gravity seems to increase for many people as they get older, making it all the more crucial to focus on standing straight and tall. A simple and effective method to develop good posture is to imagine you are suspended by a string attached to the crown of your head, like a puppet. This is the posture that keeps your head, spine, and body properly aligned. Keep your shoulders squared, your abdominal muscles firm and tight, and your head back and centered between your shoulders. Your weight should be evenly distributed on your two feet, your knees should be slightly bent, and your hips should be level.

Good posture does more than just signal good health; it can also affect the aging process. The correct posture helps maintain bone strength and joint health. Exercises to strengthen the abs will keep your lumbar spine properly aligned, as will focusing on good posture. A strong, straight trunk in correct posture fosters a natural, relaxed gait and can help to put the youthful spring back in your step. A shuffling, stooped, and slow gait will make a person look older and less attractive regardless of age. Strength and flexibility exercises are critically important for maintaining good posture and a healthy musculoskeletal system. Weight training and yoga are indispensable tools not just for delaying aging, but also for actually reversing many of its manifestations.

Julie Gudmestad, writing in the October 2004 issue of *Yoga Journal,* discussed the two most common postural problems today: 1) a hunched upper back (kyphosis), usually associated with jutting forward of the head; and 2) an extreme sway in the lower back (lordosis). These abnormal curvatures of the spine create many of the serious back problems that cause such pain and disability in America today. The excessive forward curve of the lumbar spine in lordosis pushes the abdomen forward, creating or accentuating the look of a potbelly. It also places unnatural stresses on the disks, ligaments, and bones of the lumbar spine, which is the most common place for serious back problems to develop. Weakness of the abdominal muscles is the usual cause of this sway back.

Your mother was right—you will look great and feel better if you stand up straight and tall instead of slouching. Since much of our life is spent slouched behind a steering wheel or slumped in front of a screen, you can become permanently slouched and round-shouldered. Physically active cultures do not have the epidemic of spine problems that we suffer here in the United States and in other highly mechanized modern cultures.

Many of us need to relearn how to stand and sit in a manner that supports the natural curves of the spine. To properly align yourself vertically in a standing position, concentrate on keeping your ears directly over your shoulders, your shoulders over your hips, the hips over the knees, the knees over the ankles. This little exercise may sound ridiculously simple, but stand up and give it a try. At first, you may have to frequently remind yourself consciously to practice good posture, but with time, that droopy, sagging stance will be replaced with a straight, strong bearing. When you are seated, concentrate on sitting up straight. If you are working at a screen, make sure it is not more than a few inches below eye level so you don't have to slouch over. Your sleep habits also can play an important role in maintaining or restoring good posture. Use only one pillow and try to sleep on your side without pulling your head forward into the fetal position. Avoid sleeping on your stomach, since this can aggravate back problems by accentuating an excessive forward sway in the lumbar spine.

Posture tip: Our friend Corey Scott, a bright, energetic personal trainer, encourages his clients to try sitting on a fitness ball about two feet in diameter sometimes, instead of their comfy desk chairs. Sitting on a fitness ball forces you to stabilize your body with your trunk muscles, which will automatically cause you to sit up straight. In contrast, the typical cushy C-shaped desk chair encourages a slouching posture. When you sit on a fitness ball, your thighs should be about parallel to the floor so that your knees are bent at an angle of about 90 degrees with your feet flat on the floor. Try it—you will be amazed to find that sometimes using a fitness ball for a desk chair can help to promote good posture and a build a strong core and back without even trying.

A great way to improve your posture and flexibility and keep your spine healthy is to incorporate strength training and yoga into your exercise routine. We recommend at least thirty minutes of strength training two or three times weekly and twenty to thirty minutes of yoga two to four times weekly. Please refer to the following two chapters for additional details.

12

EXERCISE:
THE FOUNTAIN
OF YOUTH

It appears that the human genome contains only 25,000 genes, or about one-third more than the lowly roundworm. Geneticists were initially surprised that something as complex as a human being could be built from such a limited blueprint. However, it is also becoming increasingly clear that gene regulation is far more important than simply the number of genes. Each gene can function in a variety of different ways depending upon how it is regulated. Perhaps the single most powerful way to regulate your genetic expression is with regular exercise. Over half of all of your genes are modified by regular physical activity. This means when you exercise regularly you literally change your genetic makeup and favorably alter almost every aspect of your being, including your appearance, body composition, mood, memory, sleep, blood pressure, hormones, and longevity. Exercise changes your genetic function, which in turn sends chemical signals that remake you into the lean, powerful, energetic, and optimistic person you were designed to be.

Many of the health problems blamed on aging are actually symptoms of deteriorating fitness and waning strength caused by idleness and apathy. Fortunately, getting back to a very physically active lifestyle will send growth and repair signals throughout your body and brain, allowing you to grow younger.

Even those of us who study physical fitness professionally have been surprised at the power of daily exercise. The fact is, it may be the single best "drug" for many health problems. It will improve cholesterol profiles by lowering the bad fats and raising the protective HDL level. Exercise will lower blood pressure and is the most effective weapon against obesity. Studies show that permanent weight loss is almost impossible without regular exercise.

With an appropriate regimen of physical activity and diet some patients with high blood pressure are able to discontinue their medications. Recent studies showed that an aerobic and strength-training exercise program, coupled with a healthy Mediterranean diet, was effective in preventing two out of three cases of diabetes.

Regular physical activity not only improves your physical strength and appearance, it also makes you feel good. A recent study tracked 174 previously sedentary men and women between the ages of sixty and seventy-five who participated in a supervised walking and stretching program. After exercising at least three times a week for six months, the participants showed significant improvements in self-esteem and reduced rates of depression. Six months after completing the program, participants who went back to a sedentary lifestyle showed deterioration in self-esteem and mood.

Never Too Late to Benefit from Exercising

In a study published in Circulation *in September 2004, investigators reported that continuous bed rest for three weeks was as detrimental to the heart and overall health as three decades of aging. The second aspect of the study showed that nothing turned back the clock on aging like regular exercise. Study participant Jim Hawkins, a seventy-one-year-old retired navy flight engineer, found that after three months of daily exercise the flexibility of his heart was restored to normal and his overall cardiac function was restored to the level of a healthy thirty-seven-year-old.*

The same chemicals (serotonin, norepinephrine, and endorphins) that become elevated in the brain in response to alcohol, tobacco, or drugs also rise immediately after exercise in people who work out regularly. In other words, it's possible to get hooked on exercise instead of harmful mood-altering chemicals. The problem is, this habit takes approximately four to eight weeks of daily workouts to develop. To remain motivated once you start exercising, try pairing up with an exercise partner (a dog is often the most available, willing, and enthusiastic partner), keeping an exercise diary, or finding new and interesting activities and places to do your workouts.

Do you feel like your battery is wearing down? In this hectic world you're not alone. Stress, sleep disorders, fatigue, and depression are among the most common complaints of Americans today. Most people have hunches about why they are always tired, but few recognize one of the main reasons: lack of exercise.

Because we're always rushing around, often under emotional pressure and deadlines, we feel as though we're being active. But the fact is jumping to conclusions, pulling your hair out, pushing papers, and climbing the wall don't quality as good exercises. All the tensions of the day leave you emotionally exhausted, and though you might think exercise is the last thing you need, it is *the best way* to recharge your battery.

When it comes to fitness, good intentions are not enough. Recently I asked one of my patients, "How often do you exercise?" He replied, "I try to work out twice a day." I responded, "Wow, that's great. How often do you actually get to it?" He said, "About once a month." Paying your monthly dues at your local fitness club will do nothing for you unless you actually do some exercise.

Family obligations, work, and sedentary habits like plopping down in front of the TV after dinner usually push exercise so far down the "to-do" list that it rarely gets done. But daily exercise should be among your top priorities. If it isn't, all the other activities that are displacing it will eventually suffer.

In time, the atrophy and disease that result from a sedentary lifestyle will leave you unfit, depressed, and in many ways, disabled. Where there's a will there's a way: If you can grasp the importance of exercise in your life, you can and will make the time for it. The best way to do this is to make it a daily habit, like brushing your teeth. Every day you need to think: "Have I gotten my exercise in?" If the answer is no, you must make a point of finding the time to do it.

If you think you're too tired for exercise, think again. Ironically, the best way to *have* more energy is to *spend* more energy exercising daily. The more fit you are, the less work it takes to accomplish any task. On the other hand, *when you quit doing the hard things your life doesn't become easier. Instead, the easy things become hard as your fitness deteriorates.* If you're having a difficult time climbing stairs, the solution is not to quit doing it, but rather to work on your strength and fitness. This strategy is essential if you want avoid the age-related loss of physical capabilities. Exercise is difficult at first, but the more you do it, the easier it becomes. After about six weeks of daily exercise you will find yourself actually looking forward to your workouts. At this point it becomes easier to think about staying fit as a permanent component of your lifestyle.

A recent study from the University of California showed that 86 percent of Americans are not getting enough exercise. This report was based on about 7,500 men and women, and it found that the top three ways people eighteen years of age and older expended energy were driving (11 percent of daily activity), doing office work (9 percent), and watching TV or movies (8.6 percent). By comparison, the top leisure-time physical activity, walking, accounted for only 1 percent of energy expenditure. If you are wondering why the average American is overweight and out of shape, it is simply because the activities that occupy most of our waking hours are driving, office work, and watching TV. Think about it—this is not conducive to good physical or mental health.

"Just no time!"—the default excuse for an inactive lifestyle—does not hold up under scrutiny. These same people watch an average of three to four hours of TV per day. Time is an issue for almost all of us today, but the president of the United States and most of your favorite screen stars are among the busiest people in the world, and yet they find the time to exercise regularly. You can, too. For most Americans, the time is there—it's the energy and the will that are usually lacking. And this is a self-perpetuating quagmire—you will not have the energy and enthusiasm for exercise until you get fit, and you can't get fit because you do not have the energy to exercise. This is your life; if you want live it to the fullest, you must make the commitment to exercise daily. You may have better luck with multiple short sessions of low-level exercise if you are having trouble finding the time and energy for physical activities at first. As your stamina and fitness improve, you will find it easier to ramp up the duration and intensity of your workout.

The latest guidelines on diet and exercise recently released by the Department of Health and Human Services call for thirty to ninety minutes of exercise daily.

This report was met with a collective sigh from the American public. What could the government possibly be thinking in recommending such an unreasonable goal for the average American? Well, the report is actually just stating the scientific evidence that shows many people need at least forty-five minutes of activity per day to keep their weight under control and prevent many of the most common diseases that are plaguing Americans today. With two-thirds of us overweight or obese and only one-third meeting the minimum goal of thirty minutes of daily exercise, it appears we just need to stop whining and start moving. How do you know if you need thirty or sixty or ninety minutes of exercise daily? Studies show that thirty minutes will give you many health benefits, but if excess weight is your problem, you will probably need sixty or ninety minutes a day. Many exercise enthusiasts like us find that they feel better with two shorter workouts on most days.

The inertia of a sedentary lifestyle is the most difficult obstacle to overcome in developing a regular fitness program. You may think you don't have the strength or energy to get some exercise, but if you just get out there and take the first step, you will begin to feel better in a matter of a few minutes. Don't think that exercise has to be uncomfortable to be beneficial. You don't have to go for the "burn"; just go for a walk. Studies show that walking at a brisk but comfortable pace will raise your heart rate to about 55 percent of its peak, which will burn calories, improve mood and cardiovascular fitness, and decrease both weight and risk of diabetes.

A recent study showed that even brief bouts of exertion that add up over the course of a day are as good as one longer episode of continuous exercise. Research has also found that getting exercise through daily activities (such as walking for nearby errands, climbing stairs, doing your daily chores with more intensity) is as good as exercising in the form of sports.

Are You 100 Percent Fit?

A landmark study published in the *New England Journal of Medicine* in 2002 studied fitness as a predictor of survival. The researchers followed a group of over 6,000 people for six years and found that next to age, the best predictor of survival was simply how fit they were as determined by a treadmill test. The longer they could go on the treadmill, the lower their risk of dying. This was more predictive than all other variables, including their family history, cholesterol and blood pressure levels, or whether or not they smoked. The bottom line is, perhaps the most important thing you can do to ensure a long life is simply to get and stay fit.

Exercise is important, but your degree of fitness is even more important. Scientists have recently come up with fitness goals that will tell you how fit you are, or ought to be, for your age. A MET (short for metabolic equivalent) is how much energy you are expending. One MET is approximately how much energy you burn while sitting quietly. As the intensity of the workout increases, your MET level increases; a casual walk is about three to six METs, running will bring take the level to ten METs or higher. Most aerobic exercise equipment these days will display the number of METs you are achieving during a workout. The table below displays data from a study published in the *New England Journal of Medicine* in August 2005. It shows how many METs you should be able to reach to be considered fit. You only need to be capable of reaching this level momentarily, not sustaining it for a prolonged period. The recent study showed that those who were able to achieve these fitness goals had a much lower risk of death from any cause.

GOAL NUMBER OF METS NEEDED TO ACHIEVE 100 PERCENT FITNESS LEVEL		
Age	Women 100 percent fitness	Men 100 percent fitness
25	11.4	11.9
30	10.8	11.4
35	10.1	10.8
40	9.5	10.3
45	8.8	9.7
50	8.2	9.2
55	7.5	8.6
60	6.9	8.1
65	6.2	7.5
70	5.6	7.0
75	4.9	6.4

How to start an exercise program:

1. *Begin slowly. Be careful not to overdo it. Do only five or ten minutes of exercise at first, even if it is only walking around the block.*

2. *Find activities that you truly enjoy. Your chances of sticking with an unpleasant program for the long term are not good.*

3. *Increase your workout time and intensity not more than about 10 percent per week.*

4. *Listen to your body. If a joint or muscle begins to hurt, ease off or find another activity to do instead for a few days. If you feel strong, go a little further or harder.*

5. *Find an exercise partner. A dog is ideal, but a friend or family member will do fine as well.*

6. *Stay well hydrated.*

7. *Get advice from a pro. Hire a personal trainer to give you pointers on what is best for you. Even if it is for only an occasional hour to receive tips and a fresh workout routine, professional input can really keep you on track.*

8. *Cross-train. This is one of the most important features of a ideal exercise routine. Different activities will prevent injuries and burnout and keep you enthused and optimally fit.*

9. *Start your exercise session slowly, with five or ten minutes at a low-level intensity warm-up pace. Save the stretching for after the exercise session. Stretching after exercise does you more good than stretching before.*

10. *Set goals and reward yourself when you achieve them. Sign up for a race or an active vacation for which you will need to train.*

ACTIVITY GUIDE TO BURNING CALORIES	
Activity	Total Calories Used per Hour
Cooking	185–200
Walking slowly (2.5 mph)	210–230
Cleaning	235–355
Brisk walking (4 mph)	250–345
Golf (walking, not riding in the golf cart)	300–350
Jogging (6 mph)	315–480
Cycling (9 mph)	315–480
Tennis	315–480
Skating	320–400
Gardening (heavy)	450–525
Basketball	480–625
Aerobic dancing	480–625
Swimming	480–625
Cross-country skiing	480–625

Go Outside and Play with Your Friends

If this phrase strikes a resonant chord in your soul and brings a smile to your face, you are not alone. Most of us heard this simple command from our parents as children. In many respects, it epitomizes the joy of youth and harkens us back to a time when we were filled with camaraderie and curiosity about the natural wonders around us.

That joy of movement, appreciation of the beauty in everyday nature, and love for fun and friendship are still a part of us. But as adults, somehow we become numb and callused, chronically relegating playtime to the back burner as more "important" matters dominate our existence.

Our capacity to reconnect with that childish, innocent love of play, nature, and friendship is inside us waiting to be rekindled. And here's the bonus—when you become more active, you don't neglect important matters. You deal with them more efficiently and energetically as you become fit and reenergized.

For most of the patients we see professionally, health concerns alone are not enough to keep them motivated to exercise frequently. On the other hand, if they realize that they will feel and look better when they get their daily exercise, they are more likely to make it a permanent part of their lifestyle. In other words, to look like a fit athlete, you have to act like one. If exercise is not something you prefer to do, your ticket to fitness is play.

Becoming and staying fit can be an opportunity to spend time with the significant people in your life. If you find an activity that you can share with friends or family, you may find yourself looking forward to your workout as a highlight of your day. Make social plans with your friends and family that center around fun physical activities. Instead of going to a movie or watching TV, plan a walk in the park with a friend or get out for a bike ride. You will burn 300 to 450 calories per hour of physical activity depending on what you choose to do. Physical play is a great way to forge friendships and strengthen interpersonal bonds. Even laughing hard for about a minute will double your heart rate for another minute or so afterward. A hearty laugh actually exercises the muscles throughout your chest and abdomen, neck, face, and scalp, and gives the heart and lungs a mini-workout. Perhaps more importantly, laughter helps lower stress hormones and blood pressure and improves immune function.

If you can play with friends while you exercise, you won't just make your life longer, you will make it fuller, happier, and more vigorous. So quit making excuses—go outside and play with your friends!

Although Joan is disciplined about working out on her stair-climber, James thinks stationary exercise is a masochistic life-extension strategy: After trudging along for what feels like about an hour and a half, he checks his watch and discovers that only ten minutes have actually elapsed. No wonder most Americans are sedentary—James would be, too, if his only option was indoor stationary exercise. He needs to feel exhilarated when he exercises, so he almost always goes outside to play. He even enjoys going out in bad weather because experiencing the different moods of nature provides a stimulating change in the routine. If this approach appeals to you, try it out! Leave the gym behind and find a way to play outside.

Play as Though Your Life Depended Upon It

When the snow flies in Kansas City, we head to the hills—to sled. As a child growing up in the extreme northeast corner of North Dakota (the coldest spot in the lower forty-eight states), James learned to have fun in the snow. Now, when the snow covers the grass completely, we have a blizzard party. We bundle up, grab the sleds and snowboards, and hurry over to a long, steep grass-covered slope the kids call Suicide Hill. For an hour or two we careen down, and scramble back up the hill, over and over again. Later, we sit around the fireplace with a cup of hot cocoa and though we are physically exhausted and a little bruised, we are a happy and relaxed bunch. Play is perhaps the most underrated element in physical fitness—its benefits are unparalleled. Active playing will confer the same or better benefits as laborious exercise: enhanced cardiopulmonary fitness, better strength and endurance, more flexibility, and improved balance and coordination. But play also bestows a sense of joy and delight—something that even an exercise addict like James would not associate with a mind-numbing forty-minute slog on a treadmill or stationary bicycle.

The workaholic American motto tells us: Work is for adults; play is for kids. Don't buy into it. Play is one of the real joys of life, and you can be playful no matter what your age. In his enlightened book *Play as If Your Life Depends on It*, Frank Forencich writes, "Because so many of our exercise programs are inherently monotonous, many exercisers go looking for motivation. It's curious that we should need so much stimulation for something that is supposedly natural. We need external motivation because the common exercise program consists of dull, laborious repetitions; in other words, work. Imagine if our exercise programs were more play-centric. The power of play lies in the fact that it gives us instant pleasurable feedback. We play because it feels good and because it feels good, we want to play more."

Fun and Practical

If A is success in life, then A = x + y + z.
Work is x, y is play, and z is keeping your mouth shut.
—ALBERT EINSTEIN

Play, like beauty, is a very subjective concept. If it is fun for you, it's play. Many people like tennis, golf, basketball, squash, or racquetball. Or you may like to go and play with your friends at the swimming pool, an aerobics class, or a yoga session. Our family loves to play in the mountains and on the beaches. Many people love to dance, which is an ideal way to play yourself into shape. On a beautiful day, there is nothing like taking kids or friends or dogs or all of the above to a wide-open place to play catch with an Aerobie. An Aerobie, a twenty-first-century version of a Frisbee, is an aerodynamic rubber ring about fourteen inches in diameter that can easily be thrown hundreds of feet. You can find one at any toy store for about ten dollars. Invite someone to go play Aerobie at a park, and you will be amazed at how much fun and exercise you get without even thinking about it. You do not have to be skilled at whatever physical endeavor you find pleasure in doing. If you are having fun, you know you are doing it right. So find activities that you enjoy and make it a priority to do something physical every day.

Sitting Ourselves to Death

We are hard-wired to prefer sitting and resting rather than doing physical work. Our ancestors needed to rest whenever possible to preserve their strength and energy for the daily rigors of securing their food, water, and protection. James always asks his patients, "Do you have any unusual symptoms like chest pressure when you physically exert yourself?" They often respond, "I never exert myself." Today, modern technology has engineered our world to be ultraconvenient so that we can indeed go through life without ever having to do any strenuous physical exertion. If you are going to be vigorous, attractive, and healthy in contemporary America, you will have to do something that might feel uncomfortable and unnatural, especially at first: *move and exert yourself just for the sake of exercise.* After you overcome your inertia and do some vigorous activity, you can perceive the immediate benefits to your mental and physical well-being, and you can recognize that this was exactly what your body needed.

Suggestions to Help You Succeed in Exercising Consistently

Walk or run in your neighborhood or during coffee or lunch breaks at your worksite. You will burn about the same number of calories per mile whether you stroll, walk, or run, although higher intensity activities will improve fitness faster and more effectively and also rev up your metabolism so you will burn more calories even while at rest. Find an exercise partner, or get a dog. Set goals like entering an upcoming fun walk or run. Exercise hard enough to break a sweat to be sure you are building cardiovascular fitness. Another good rule of thumb on exercise intensity is that you should be able to carry on a conversation while exercising, though not as effortlessly as when you are standing still.

Stress: Fighting the Enemy Within

For millennia, physical exercise wasn't an option—it was a necessity. Fitness wasn't a special trait reserved for the motivated and energetic members of the tribe. Even the meek gatherers developed endurance and strength as they traveled the grasslands and carried food and water back to camp. Obesity or weakness were usually fatal. In essence, Stone Age humans were either fit or they were dead.

Today, we face very different kinds of stress. Starvation, predators, life-and-death physical confrontations with hostile strangers, and serious prolonged exposure to extreme cold or heat are all thankfully absent from our day-to-day lives. Instead, most of our stress is in the form of anxiety, fear, and worries about abstract threats such as overwhelming financial obligations, interpersonal conflicts, work deadlines, taxes, risk of diseases, and the like. Our systems react to these modern stresses as if a physical response was required to survive them. But higher blood pressure and faster pulse and increased cortisol, glucose, and adrenaline levels do nothing to help us come up with the money to pay overdue bills.

When the hunter-gatherer occasionally encountered a major stress, his blood surged with powerful hormones that mobilized his system for action. He ran or fought with heightened intensity and effectively flushed these hormones and chemicals from his system. Imagine his version of day-to-day anxiety: "It was terrifying. I had speared a small deer and was bringing it home when a pack of wolves surrounded me. I thought they were going to kill me. I was so frightened that my mind was racing, my heart was pounding, my palms were sweaty, and my hands were quivering with fear. I dropped the deer and ran for my life. By the time I finally made it back to camp, I was exhausted; but now I've settled down, and I feel fine."

Compare that stressful experience with the typical stress encountered by the persistently harassed modern American. "Monday morning I received an e-mail from my boss telling me that the company is downsizing my department by 25 percent and to expect layoffs over the next year. I don't know what would happen if I lost my job now. Our credit cards are maxed out; we have a huge house payment every month, and three kids to support with hardly anything in our savings. That afternoon the doctor's office called to tell me my PSA is mildly elevated, and I might need a biopsy. All I can think about is how my grandfather suffered with prostate cancer. I feel like my life is just unraveling; my heart has been pounding, my fingers and toes are cold. All week I haven't been able to sleep, and I am just stressed out. I know I should exercise, but I just don't have the time with all my deadlines at work and responsibilities at home."

Stresses today rarely present immediate physical threats, yet your brain instinctively mobilizes your systems to prepare as if you will have to fight or run for your life. To make matters worse, many of these stresses linger both in reality and in our imagined fears, and it doesn't take much for many people to switch on the stress response—an argument with your spouse, or a looming job deadline, for example. They can be corrosive and eventually will wear down your immunity and leave you emotionally exhausted. This sort of unrelenting anxiety renders us vulnerable to chronic diseases like high blood pressure, diabetes, heart disease, depression, and even cancer. The Paleolithic hunter naturally and quickly cleansed the stress chemicals from his system with vigorous exercise and grew stronger and faster because of it. The modern worried and overweight warrior just stews in his own juices, wearing himself down without realizing that the real enemy lies within.

Despite what most people believe, stress is not the real problem today, nor is it the body's automatic stress response. It is the never-ending nature of the stress that drains your health and vitality plus the fact that it is not accompanied by vigorous physical activity. When the world feels like it is closing in around you, move—not just to the refrigerator or the vending machine—go out and get some exercise! When you come home from your brisk walk, weight-lifting session, or jog, you will be able to put your worries in perspective and get back to living an enjoyable and productive life.

What Is the Best Time of Day to Exercise?

Joan insists this is when James rolls out of bed each morning, puts on his running shoes or in-line skates, and takes our two border collies out for a run. She finds this keeps the dogs and James more relaxed and easier to live with for the rest of the day. We have found that most people seem to be able to comply with a morning exercise routine best. Studies done by Dr. Art Mollen compared the time of day that exercise was performed with the likelihood of long-term compliance to the program. He found that after one year about 75 percent of people who started a morning exercise regimen were still exercising. Of those who chose a noontime routine, 50 percent were following the program. If his patients waited till the end of the day to exercise, only about 25 percent were still complying with the exercise program one year later.

An easy way to increase your body's ability to burn fat is to exercise before you eat breakfast. When you work out first thing in the morning before eating, you force your body to mobilize fat stores for fuel. Whether it is walking, jogging, cycling, or weight lifting, when you attack your body fat first, you get to your goal weight sooner—as an added bonus, you accomplish your workout at the start of your day.

This Is Your Brain. This Is Your Brain on Exercise

If the improvements in weight, mood, and appearance aren't enough of an incentive to exercise, maybe the knowledge that your brain is at stake will motivate you to get moving. The link between physical exercise and brain health has been clearly established. Scientific studies consistently show that regular cardiovascular conditioning improves memory, delays aging and shrinkage of the brain, and lowers the risk of Alzheimer's disease. Dr. Dharma Singh Khalsa, author of *Brain Longevity,* states, "What is good for the heart is good for the head." Exercise has been shown even to increase the growth of new brain cell branches, effectively improving your brain power. A thirty-minute sessioin of aerobic exercise resuls in an immediate improvement in your ability to process complex information. An intense cardio workout has been estimated to sharpen mental focus just as well as a dose of ADD (attention deficit disorder) medication.

The brain-protective benefits of regular exercise were demonstrated in a study by Dr. Robert Friedland and colleagues. They found that people who had been getting regular exercise from age twenty to sixty were three times less likely to develop Alzheimer's disease later in life. The brain protection was noted for a wide range of activities, including gardening and other physical endeavors not done purely for the sake of obtaining exercise. Another study by Dr. Arthur Kramer found that subjects who did more physical conditioning during their life showed less age-related shrinkage in brain size compared to that noted in sedentary people. Science shows that athletes in their sixties or older have better reaction times and quicker mental responses compared to inactive people of similar ages. The older athletes also outperformed their sedentary contemporaries in measurements of memory, attention, intelligence, and reasoning. Although speculative at this point, it is likely that exercise improves blood vessel health, resulting in better delivery of oxygen and nutrients to brain tissues and also possibly improves hormones and reduces stress levels.

Dr. Gary Small, neurologist and author, did a study to evaluate the effects of an optimal diet and lifestyle (very similar to the Forever Young plan) on the functioning of the brain. He did a baseline PET scan on the brain to assess how well it was functioning before the start of the program. The study individuals were then randomized to a healthy diet that was high in nutrients, low in calories, reduced in sugar and other processed carbs, high in omega-3 fats, but low in bad fats such as saturated fats and trans fats. The subjects were also started on aerobic exercises, relaxation techniques, and brain teasers (crossword puzzles, etc.). By the end of the trial, the subjects following the program showed a substantial improvement in their brain functioning by PET scan, especially in the prefrontal cortex, the area that is associated with working memory, stress, and anxiety. Not surprisingly, the study patients also had a ten point drop in their blood pressure and significant weight loss.

Walking: America's Favorite Exercise

America is now the fattest nation in the world. We also have the lowest percentage of daily outings done on foot. Over the last two decades, trips Americans made by bicycling and walking declined by about 50 percent. This dramatic drop in physical movement disturbed the fundamental energy balance equation: Calories taken in should equal calories burned. We're eating more, yet exercising less—a lot less.

Before the advent of the automobile and other modern conveniences, Americans didn't worry much about keeping fit. Who needs to work out when you spend your day reaping and sowing, lifting and carrying, pounding and sawing—all by hand? Researchers at the University of Tennessee studied a group of Old Order Amish to try to put our society's lack of movement in perspective. These people shun cars and other modern conveniences, and thus provide clues to the activity patterns of bygone generations. The researchers outfitted the Amish with pedometers and found that the average Amish man took over 18,000 steps a day, and the average woman over 14,000 steps a day. In contrast, the typical modern American takes 5,000 steps a day.

Still, when it comes to the preferred form of exercise, walking wins hands down. Almost 80 million Americans are recreational walkers; 15 million of them classify as serious fitness walkers—someone who walks for fitness two or more times weekly. What makes walking so popular? For starters it's convenient, it takes no special skills or practice, it's safe, and it's easy and fun to walk with friends. We love it because walking provides a myriad of health perks.

Vigorous exercise, like stair-climbing, running, full-court basketball, or cross-country skiing will develop fitness and burn off body fat with workouts of shorter duration (as little as fifteen to thirty minutes daily). The intensity of your workout matters tremendously. When it comes to any form of exercise, it is quality not quantity that counts most. A 145-pound person jogging at a ten minutes per mile pace (a speed of six miles per hour) for thirty minutes will burn off about 350 calories. The same person walking at a seventeen minutes per mile pace (three and a half miles per hour) will have to walk one hour and fifteen minutes to burn the same number of calories. If you are on a tight time schedule, make the exercise session short but strenuous. We often find that knowing we have only twenty or thirty minutes to exercise imparts an urgency to the workout that cranks up the intensity to a higher level than if we are not pressed for time. Even if we have only twenty or thirty minutes, we often get out for a quick run, go down to the basement for a brisk weight workout, or even go for a fast bike ride or skate around the neighborhood.

Walking is good exercise, but walking briskly is even better. Although it is great to progress from a leisurely to a moderate to hard pace, exercising to extremely difficult levels does not provide further cardiovascular protection and can predispose you to injuries and even heart attack and sudden death. For most people a brisk walk is about four miles per hour, or a fifteen-minute mile. Three miles an hour, or a twenty-minute mile is a light to moderate pace, and two miles per hour is a stroll.

Try to avoid walking on concrete when you can. Humans were not designed to walk and run predominantly on rock surfaces, and this eventually takes a toll on your musculoskeletal system. Walking or running on natural surfaces like grass, dirt, gravel, or mulch is much healthier for your joints. Other joint-friendly options include composite track surfaces, treadmills, and stair-climbers. Good shoes, with excellent support and cushioning, are important as well. Old broken-down shoes can lead to old broken-down joints. If you run or walk on a track, make sure you are not always walking the same direction, since that can lead to strain and injury of knee and hip joints. If you want to rejuvenate your life with walking, you need to be like President Harry Truman. "Give 'em hell Harry" attributed his irrepressible, energetic, and optimistic lifestyle to his daily walk. When President Truman left the house, he always stepped out with a purpose. "Walking as if I had someplace important to be," as he put it. Even when he was retired with nothing more urgent to do than hike to downtown Independence, Missouri, to chat with friends and pick up a newspaper, he kept up his brisk pace. It kept Harry fit, sharp, and spunky for almost nine decades despite having to deal with some pretty formidable stresses—it can do the same for you.

What's the goal? If you are just getting started, shoot for about thirty minutes three to four times weekly at three to four mph (twenty and fifteen minutes per mile respectively). If you are trying to lose weight you will have to do more, about forty-five to sixty minutes at least three or four times each week, maintaining a pace of approximately three and a half to four and a half mph. Those of you who are targeting improved cardiovascular fitness should be building up to four to five mph or faster as your fitness improves and you become comfortable with a quicker pace. Your goal is to perform a heavy-breathing, sweat-producing, twenty-to-forty-minute exercise session three to four or more times per week. If you just cannot or will not get this done, there is another option . . . count your steps.

10K a Day

How much walking is enough? If you want the simplest state-of-the-art answer to the question of how much walking is enough, all you need to remember is "10,000 steps a day." Researchers have proven that people who walk this much each day are getting what they need to achieve aerobic fitness. Most people cover a mile in somewhere between 1,800 steps (for those with longer legs and strides) and 2,200 steps (for those with shorter strides). For the average adult 10,000 steps translates to about five miles a day.

For each 200 steps you take, you burn about ten calories. When you take an extra 2,000 steps, which translates into about one mile, you burn about 100 calories. If you gradually work up to 10,000 steps a day, you will get all the aerobic activity you need without having to worry about how far you have walked, if you walked all at once, or how much you walked intermittently throughout the day.

Most sedentary office workers take about 2,000 to 5,000 steps in a typical workday, so they need to come up with another 5,000 to 8,000 steps somewhere else. If you are really creative and conscientious about looking for opportunities to take extra steps during your day, you may not need any scheduled walking or running time. But most people will need to walk an uninterrupted two to three miles daily (4,000 to 6,000 steps). This means getting out and walking briskly for about thirty minutes sometime during the day. Be careful not to overdo it at first. If you are sedentary and getting only 1,000 to 3,000 or so steps a day and most of those steps are to the refrigerator and back during television commercials, you need to start with "baby steps." Try for 4,000 steps each day and gradually increase your daily accumulation of steps.

Initially, all this may seem entirely out of the question, but think for a moment about all the opportunities you have to walk each day. You can easily measure your steps if you have an inconspicuous digital friend who is keeping track of your efforts. A digital pedometer is a great motivational tool, and it provides concrete feedback about what you have accomplished each day. When you know you are "getting credit" for the extra effort you are making, you might find yourself walking on nearby errands, opting for the stairs more often, and taking advantage of work breaks to get some steps in. Pedometers are inexpensive, reliable, and fun. If you are serious about getting fit but can't seem to be able to find the time, get a digital pedometer.

A recent study in women showed a close relationship between the number of steps taken daily and fitness. The women taking less than 6,000 steps daily had a BMI of 29, 44 percent body fat, and a thirty-seven-inch waist. Those taking 6,000 to 10,000 steps had a BMI of 26, 35 percent body fat, and a thirty-two-inch waist. The women who averaged 10,000 or more steps per day had a BMI of 23, 26 percent body fat, and a twenty-nine-inch waist.

Climb Your Way to Fitness

James's grandmother Alice Vick was infamous for her frankness, or lack of tact, depending on your perspective. She would do things like ask the young girl with a wild hairstyle who was ringing her up at the grocery store, "Do you actually *try* to make your hair look like that?" Alice Vick's husband, the grandfather James never met, died of alcoholism as a young man, leaving her to raise four young children alone on the meager wages of a seamstress working out of a small apartment. She often said, "It's a great life if you don't weaken," referring to the importance of maintaining an optimistic but tough mental outlook. Before she died at age ninety-three, she told us she had about eighty-five good years. In fact, she never did lose her strong will and sharp wit, but it was her loss of physical strength that made the last few years of her life difficult. For decades she lived on the third floor of an apartment building in downtown Crookston, a quaint little town in the northeastern corner of Minnesota. She never owned a car, and she stayed strong by carrying her groceries up two flights of stairs in the front of her building and taking the garbage down the two flights to the back alley. She couldn't afford a taxi, so she walked virtually everywhere she wanted to go. At eighty-five, Alice decided that she could no longer climb those stairs, and she moved into a retirement apartment on the ground floor. The move precipitated a steep downward spiral in her physical strength and quality of life.

On January 30, 2005, a pair of twin sisters, Siri Ingvarsson and Gunhild Gaell-stedt, celebrated their 100 birthday. They still are physically sound and mentally sharp. The sisters have lived in the same apartment building in Stockholm, Sweden, for more than fifty years, Siri on the second floor and Gunhild on the third. The building has no elevator, and the twin sisters attribute their longevity to the fact that they have been busily scampering up and down the stairwells for half a century and still do today.

Get in the habit of taking the stairs. If you establish the routine of automatically opting for the stairwell rather than the elevator, you will take a huge step toward staying lean and fit. Modern conveniences like elevators, escalators, remote controls, dishwashers, and automatic car washes "save" you about 110 calories daily. By the time a year passes, this translates to about ten extra pounds of body fat that you are carrying around. Stair-climbing is an excellent no-gym workout—a chance to burn some calories and improve your fitness during your daily routine. It is the most vigorous physical activity most Americans do and, as a bonus, taking the stairs usually saves time compared to waiting for an elevator. Studies show that stair-climbing will burn twelve and a half calories every one minute you spend climbing up, and four calories per minute spent descending. We make a point of taking the stairs virtually all the time, unless it is a climb of more than six to ten floors. Stair-climbing not only burns calories, it also tones your legs and butt muscles.

While climbing up is a great exercise, going down burns only one-third of the calories and is more traumatic for your joints. The knees especially take a real pounding when descending stairs. The faster you descend, the more stress and strain there is on the tendons, ligaments, and cartilage of the joints. Sometimes when James is traveling and staying in a high-rise hotel, he will make several trips running up the ten or more flights, and recovering in the elevator on the way down. In only fifteen to thirty minutes he gets an awesome interval workout! However, we must warn you that you may get some funny looks from the other hotel guests as you stumble, breathless and sweaty, into the elevator.

The Rejuvenating Effects of Strength Training: Live Stronger, Better, Longer

If you want to stay young, you have to stay strong. A fundamental but highly modifiable part of the aging process is a morphing of your body shape and composition. Women, even when they are young and fit, tend to have higher body fat levels than men. The typical twenty-year-old woman has 20 percent body fat level, which increases to 30 percent by age thirty. To make matters worse, you will lose muscle mass every year over age thirty unless you do strength training. If you are forty or fifty and weigh about as much as you did when you were twenty, you probably have a lot more fat and less muscle than you did then. By the time the average woman celebrates her fiftieth birthday, almost one-half of her body weight is composed of fat. Increasing muscle mass increases basal metabolism. This helps burn calories even when you are not exercising and makes losing weight faster and easier. A forceful body will also allow you to regain the balance and coordination you had as a young adult, and that will enable you to do things that many middle-aged people give up on, like snow-skiing, mountain climbing, basketball, or singles tennis. Additionally, weight lifting is, unquestionably, the quickest way to reshape your body for a younger more attractive look.

The medical community now realizes that the best program for overall health and cardiovascular fitness includes both aerobic and strength-training components. Without weight training to maintain muscle and bone strength, many people find an aerobic exercise program difficult for long periods of time due to muscle strain or injury, arthritis, or even broken bones. In fact, if you are over sixty, strength training may be the single most important component of your exercise program.

As people get older, some leisure activities and tasks become harder to do so they give them up. By doing less and less, their loss of muscle and bone strength accelerates. Eventually, even the activities required for daily living become difficult or impossible, and the person becomes truly "old." The only way to prevent this gradual erosion is through strength-training exercises.

We believe that much of the aging process comes down to just settling for less in life. When you develop an issue like back trouble, the typical response is to accept that you can no longer do many of the activities you used to enjoy like golf, gardening, weight lifting, or waterskiing. Instead, you should be thinking, "What can I do to strengthen this weakness so that I can return to my fully functional level?"

By getting stronger and staying strong, you can break this downward spiral of aging and weakness and enjoy a more active lifestyle with an improved quality of life. Strength training is also beneficial for the heart. As the body becomes stronger, blood pressure and heart rate remain more consistent, and you will find that daily activities such as carrying a child or a bag of groceries are easier. Furthermore, with strength training, the muscle mass increases and the amount of fat decreases. These changes improve cholesterol and blood sugar levels. Building lean body mass also will increase your metabolism, allowing you to burn more calories even at rest. Strength training influences the way your brain regulates hunger and seems to leave you less susceptible to junk food cravings. In men, a good weight-training session will increase testosterone levels over the ensuing forty-eight hours. This helps to improve mood and maintain vitality and vigor.

Starting a strength-training exercise program, especially for patients with heart disease, is best done in a supervised setting. Most health clubs have strength-training equipment and trained personnel instructors to coach members in its proper use. Physical therapists can also help design a strength program.

Seven Benefits of Weight Lifting

1. *Makes daily activities such as carrying children, lifting groceries, climbing stairs, and doing housework easier.*
2. *Improves mood; reduces anxiety and depression.*
3. *Reduces risk of injuries during sports and other physical activities.*
4. *Increases bone strength and improves posture.*
5. *Lowers blood pressure in the long term; improves cholesterol levels.*
6. *Improves appearance by building muscle and burning fat.*
7. *Alters hormone profile, bringing it closer to where it was at younger ages.*

Many people do better exercising in an interactive rather than an isolated environment. An audience can motivate people, especially guys. Men can use their innately competitive nature to their advantage if they sometimes work out around other exercisers. One study by Matthew Rhea, PhD, published in the *Journal of Strength and Conditioning Research*, found that men were able to bench press an average of forty-one pounds more when spectators were present than when they were lifting alone. Curves is an excellent structured program for women that is focused on strength training, something that is often neglected by females.

It is important to begin with relatively light weights—one to three pounds for each arm and three to five pounds for each leg, depending on your current level of muscular strength. You can gradually increase the weight, and within a few weeks, you will be making real progress in your strength. You should be able to lift each weight at least eight but not more than fifteen or twenty times. If you can't lift a weight eight times without stopping to rest, it is too heavy. If you can lift it more than twenty times, it is probably too light. As your strength gradually improves and lifting the weight eight to fifteen times is no longer a challenge, it is time to increase the load. However, high-repetition weight lifting is also an effective way to stay strong and toned without putting undue stress on your muscles and joints.

It is important to lift the weights relatively slowly. Each lift should take approximately seven to nine seconds: three to four seconds to raise the weight, one second to pause, and three to four seconds to lower the weight.

Heavy weights can predispose you to injury and an excessive increase in blood pressure and heart rate, which can trigger angina (heart pain) in people with blocked heart arteries. For patients with serious heart disease, it is best to begin a weight-training program only after discussing it with your cardiologist, and ideally in the setting of a cardiac rehab program. If you have an aneurysm of a blood vessel (an abdominal aortic aneurysm is the most common type) you should not start a weight-lifting program without consulting with your physician.

Life Is Not a Spectator Sport

Football combines the two worst features of American life:
violence and committee meetings.
—GEORGE WILL

We have learned to make a point of going outside to play during our local Kansas City Chiefs football games because we can count on having the parks and roads pretty much to ourselves for those three or four hours. One recent Indian summer Sunday, we visited a friend's cabin on Linn Valley Lake, an hour south of town. The crystal clear, smooth-as-glass lake was deserted on that gorgeous late-September day because everyone was inside watching the football game. We played all afternoon, hiking and swimming, jet-skiing, and pulling the kids on a tube behind the boat. As we made our way back into town relaxed and laughing, we noticed everyone else seemed to be unhappy and irritable. While we were having fun, the Chiefs were losing their third straight game; the opponent's last-second field goal ruined an otherwise glorious day for all those who devoted the afternoon to watching others play.

Quit Watching and Start Living:
Turn the TV, DVD, and Computer Off

> In the game of life, even seats on the fifty-yard line don't interest me.
> I came to play.
> —H. JACKSON BROWN

At point A, you are delivered into this wonderful world squinting and screaming and full of potential. At point B, you are history. What you do with those 30,000 (plus or minus a few thousand) days is up to you. Unfortunately, television is a black hole into which much of your precious time disappears. You aren't going to live forever, though we sometimes get lulled into acting as though life were just a rehearsal. In many respects, your time is the most important commodity in life. Trust me, when you are on your deathbed someday, you will not be saying "If only I had watched more TV." People who are well read are often sharp and in tune with the world and are generally admired, but being "well viewed" won't do much for you except make you bored and overweight. You burn more calories on an hourly basis sleeping than you do channel surfing with the remote. Television (like other passive screen-viewing activities) hypnotizes us into wasting a substantial proportion of our waking free time, and has become a major distraction from the real world. Often, it even intrudes upon our tranquility and inner peace. Along with movies, the computer, and the Internet, TV creates an artificial world that sets the stage for disappointment since the real world is usually not as exciting or fast moving.

> Television is important. It keeps people
> from noticing what's really going on.
> —MICHAEL BARNES

Rather than experiencing the lasting richness and fullness of reality, many Americans settle for a meaningless mock-up that robs them of time and leaves them with little to nothing to show for it. Your life is defined by the choices you make. A study published in April 9, 2003, issue of the *Journal of the American Medical Association* found that your chances of being obese go up 23 percent for every two hours of TV viewing per day, and they go down 24 percent for every one hour of exercise per day. The answer to your weight problem is as simple as turning off the TV and going outside to play.

Don't get us wrong, the TV is often on around the O'Keefe household, and occasionally we do sit down at the end of the day to watch it for a few minutes. Television is one way to relax after a long day, and the Internet will continue to revolutionize our lives for decades to come. Excess viewing, however, is a vicious cycle whereby the more you watch the more you weigh and the less energy you have and the more sedentary you become.

Our philosophy is to save TV and computer time for the day when our options are limited—when we are too old or debilitated to go out and play, enjoy a romantic evening, or climb a mountain and watch the clouds sail overhead. When we have to settle for a vicarious life, we will. Until then, we don't care if we ever see another television program. Do it, don't just watch it. Life is short.

Everybody Dies, but Not Everybody Lives

> A ship is safe in the harbor, but that is not what ships are made for.
> —ADMIRAL GRACE HOPPER

Although we live in a safer, more comfortable, affluent world today, the incidence of depression is at an all-time high. Many of us, particularly males, feel the need to take some risks to stay enthused and invigorated. Last summer James went hiking in France with Evan, Jimmy, and several of their teenage friends. One day, they trekked fifteen miles on trails that ran along the spectacular cliffs abutting the Mediterranean coast. These *calanques*, as they are they are called by the French, tower dramatically over the sea, sometimes plummeting vertically over 1,000 feet to the water below. At the midpoint of the hike from La Ciotat to Cassis and back, they found some cliffs just as sheer though not quite so high. As it turned out, this was an ideal spot for cliff-jumping—a favorite sport among the local young men who jump or even dive from heights as high as eighty feet into the deep blue sea below.

Of course, Jimmy and his buddies insisted on doing some cliff-jumping of their own. After a few leaps into the churning ocean forty-five feet below, Jimmy and his wide-eyed friends insisted that James give it a go. As he stood on the ledge, James's instincts were screaming inside his head: "Don't do it!" but he did. He leaped, and it turned out to be the first of many cliff jumps that week. Though they sometimes left him a little sore the next day, they were a highlight of the trip. Flying through the air and splashing into the refreshing crystal-clear salt water was an addictive rush that left them recharged and energized.

Mario Andretti said, "If everything seems under control, you aren't going fast enough." Our experience tells us that taking an occasional calculated risk is a great way to revitalize one's outlook and remind us that we are alive and well. Of course, we don't mean putting yourself in harm's way, like using cocaine, practicing unsafe sex, driving drunk, smoking, or not wearing seat belts. There are many reasonably safe, exhilarating adventures you can try: parasailing, bike racing, scuba diving, surfing, rock climbing, ocean swimming, paintballing, white-water rafting, snowskiing, or snowboarding are just a few. While we don't encourage taking undue risks, we do support novelty to keep you motivated and enthused about staying physically active. Even traveling to new places and meeting new people can get you out of your rut and fired up again. We like to think of life itself as a great adventure that we need to train for to fully participate in and enjoy. An upcoming journey or event is an excellent motivational tool for getting back into shape.

13

FLEXIBILITY, BREATHING, AND YOGA

Yoga and several related disciplines like t'ai chi and Pilates are among the fastest growing activities on the American fitness scene, and for good reason. Yoga is great for increasing flexibility and strength, and it also induces a sense of calm and well-being. These stretches involve the use of various poses, postures, and slow movements and are excellent techniques for improving balance and strengthening your crucially important "core" back and trunk muscles. Yoga is also excellent for keeping your spine and back strong and healthy. If you can practice these ancient fitness disciplines regularly, you will definitely notice improvements in mood, flexibility, and strength. Yoga can also improve your posture and restore ease and grace to your movement, making you feel and look younger and healthier.

Interestingly, a study from Yale presented at the American Heart Association Scientific Sessions in November 2004 also found that people who practiced yoga with meditation at least three times weekly reduced their blood pressure, pulse, and the risk of heart disease. In this study, a routine of yoga with meditation improved blood vessel function by 17 percent in healthy volunteers. However, for those with preexisting heart disease, yoga improved circulatory function by an astounding 70 percent. Yoga lowers stress and makes the blood vessels healthier and more responsive, and you don't have to be a yoga master to reap the benefits. In the Yale study, volunteers who had no prior training or experience with yoga showed dramatic improvements after following a ninety-minute yoga-meditation regimen three times weekly for six weeks. They also lowered their blood pressure from 130/79 to 125/74, with a striking reduction in the heart rate of nine beats per minute. Yoga even reduced the average weight modestly, from a BMI of 29 to 28. Recent studies show that t'ai chi is as effective as brisk walking at lowering heart rate, blood pressure, and stress hormones.

The long, slow stretches, deep breathing, and meditation of yoga won't burn calories anywhere near as well as a run on the treadmill. Yet it might be one of your best weapons to prevent the typical middle-age weight gain. A study published in the July/August 2005 issue of the journal *Alternative Therapies in Health and Medicine* found that people in their fifties who regularly practiced yoga lost about five pounds over a decade compared to a similar group that didn't do yoga who on average gained 13.5 pounds during that same time. Yoga's ability to prevent obesity probably has less to do with calorie-burning and more to do with stress relief and keeping you in tune with your body. This study involving 15,500 people found that those who practiced yoga generally avoided junk food and overeating. A yoga session will leave you feeling refreshed and relaxed, and less susceptible to mindless overeating in response to stress, boredom, depression, and the like. This is just one of the reasons we believe yoga is one of the nicest things you can do for your body and mind.

Medical scientists realize that the autonomic (involuntary) nervous system plays a key role in overall cardiovascular health. Yoga is an excellent way to improve the vagal tone (relaxation response) while at the same time reducing the fight or flight (stress) hormones. If you incorporate deep breathing techniques during your yoga sessions, you will magnify the stress reduction and autonomic nervous system benefits that help to keep your brain, cardiovascular system, and immunity youthful and strong. Yoga also improves sleep. A Harvard study found that people who followed a thirty- to forty-five-minute daily yoga routine fell asleep 30 percent faster and were awake 35 percent less during the night. Yoga lowers stress hormones and thus can improve sleep quality.

Yoga, Pilates, and t'ai chi are relatively easy to learn; just be sure to start slowly with a beginners' class and don't overdo the stretches at first. Incorporate at least one or two yoga sessions per week into your fitness routine. Either join a class to get started, or just buy or rent a yoga videotape and learn at home. By doing a variety of different types of exercise, you will be less likely to suffer boredom and burnout. Additionally, cross-training improves your overall fitness and stamina, and makes you more resistant to injury.

With nothing more than a towel or yoga mat (and even these are optional), yoga can be done almost anywhere: inside or outside, at a quiet beach, on the back patio, in your yard, or in a park. Yoga can help prevent musculoskeletal injuries and may improve the health of your immune system, which can protect you from infections and cancer. What has really fueled the rapid rise in yoga's popularity, however, is its remarkable ability to cleanse the mind of stress and worries and leave you refreshed and relaxed. You will see these improvements with your first yoga session.

About two years ago, James discovered that if he did thirty minutes of yoga in our sauna after the younger children were in bed, he slept much better and felt more energized, focused, and relaxed the next morning. Now the yoga sauna has become a ritual that he does about four nights of the week, and it has changed his life—he has no more headaches, fewer injuries during strenuous exercise, and a more centered and relaxed perspective. In summary, yoga is one of the single best things you can do to improve your long-term health and well-being.

Flexibility, the Key to Staying Young

The heart and arteries, like the mind, lose youthful elasticity with age unless you work at staying flexible. The best way to prevent stiffening of the heart is to exercise daily. A new study by the National Institutes of Health published in *Circulation* in September 2004 found that regular physical activity helps keep the heart young by preventing age-related stiffening of the cardiovascular system. The loss of suppleness begins to show up as a falloff in endurance and stamina and leads to shortness of breath. This often progresses to congestive heart failure by the time a person reaches sixty-five or seventy years of age. The normal heart is like a soft yet strong rubber band. It stretches to fill fully while it is not pumping and then snaps back during contraction to pump the blood throughout the body. Just as the skin, joints, muscles, brain, and even the eyeballs become less elastic with the passing years; your heart also becomes less flexible with age. The essence of staying young is to restore suppleness and litheness to your being.

Stretching is vitally important to staying youthful and is best done after exercise or at other times during the day. We believe that yoga is one of the best ways to develop flexibility since the stretches are held for thirty to sixty seconds while you focus on slowing and deepening your breathing. Do not bounce or force the stretches and focus on gradual progress in flexibility. Stay with a stretch and back away if you feel undue tension in a muscle or joint. Then return slowly to the stretch and gradually limber up the area. Slow stretches that are held longer (as in yoga) are the best way to improve flexibility.

Today, the old-fashioned advice to stretch before exercising is being called into question. Sure, it is still important to warm up before going full blast into any activity, particularly if you have arthritis. However, experts now agree that time spent stretching before an activity would be better spent in other ways. The ideal warm-up is to do the activity at a lower level. For example, if you are going out for a run, start with a walk, then ease into a jog, and gradually bring your pace up to full speed. This stimulates increased blood flow to the muscles involved, stretches ligaments and tendons, and safely prepares you for more forceful efforts. A recent scientific review published in the September 2004 *Clinical Journal of Sports Medicine* showed that stretching before athletic contests worsens maximal performance in activities such as weight lifting, jumping, and sprinting. Stretching before the event also does not reduce injury or soreness, and may even increase these problems. On the other hand, regular stretching done after your workouts or apart from other exercise improves athletic performance and reduces injury risk.

Why Sauna Therapy Is HOT

In college, James and his friends regularly took saunas after playing basketball. Even back then it seemed to relax and de-stress his system. He had gotten away from this habit until we moved into our current home five years ago. We bought the house from Bud, an elderly friend and patient of James's who moved to an apartment at age eighty-four after losing his wife. Bud was a remarkable man and died at eighty-nine. He was bright, witty, and engaging and looked and acted decades younger than his true age. This was always a real mystery to us because Bud was not exactly a poster boy for men's health. He smoked cigars, drank too much, paid no attention whatsoever to his diet, and although he enjoyed golf, he always rode a cart (usually stocked with stogies and beer). Still, he seemed to defy his age until the last year or two of his life.

Eventually, James discovered that Bud's daily routine involved a long hot sauna, and Bud swore that this was what kept him young and healthy. Over the past few years James has used Bud's sauna and has become a firm believer in the mental and physical benefits of sauna therapy.

The surface temperature of your skin rises quickly when you take a sauna. This stimulates sweating, which acts like a diuretic—chasing excess salt and water from your system and lowering blood pressure. Virtually all of us eat more salt than we need, and 90 percent of us are destined to develop high blood pressure during our lifetime. Therefore, this diuretic effect of sauna therapy may be an important non-pharmacologic way to keep our fluids, electrolytes, and blood pressures in healthy ranges. Amazingly, regular sauna therapy has also been shown to improve your autonomic nervous system, reducing stressful fight or flight reactions, and augmenting the relaxation response. A sauna in the evening about thirty to sixty minutes before bedtime is, in our opinion, one of the very best ways to calm your system down and ensure a sound, restful night's sleep.

The skin, our largest organ, typically eliminates about 30 percent of the body's wastes. Regular heavy sweating is a uniquely effective mechanism for ridding your body of toxic contaminants like the countless potentially harmful chemicals we ingest and breathe in each day. A study of 200 people who used a sauna regularly revealed blood chemistry changes indicating a detoxification effect induced by repeated heavy sweating. Another trial evaluating four months of regular sauna therapy showed a 40 percent reduction in toxic pesticide levels in the fat tissues of Michigan farmers. This is a unique and important effect of sweating and sauna therapy because many of these toxins are otherwise notoriously difficult to remove from storage sites like body fat.

Vigorous physical activity is another way to obtain the benefits of profuse sweating, but many people (like Bud) just don't enjoy exercise enough to do it regularly. So if you are going to be a couch potato, at least try to be a *baked* couch potato. The amount of blood pumped per minute through the cardiovascular system more than doubles during a typical sauna, much of it going to the skin in an attempt to cool it down. We suspect that this increased blood flow to the skin plays a substantial role in the antiaging effects of regular sauna that were so apparent in Bud's complexion.

The markedly increased blood flow to the skin nourishes and rejuvenates it, giving you the healthy glow of youth. This increase in blood flow is in the same range as that seen with vigorous physical activity, which is generally considered to be an essential component in any legitimate strategy to stay fit and young.

Taking a sauna regularly is a practical and effective way to reap many of the benefits of exercise without actually doing physical work. Sauna therapy increases blood flow throughout the vascular system, stimulating the vessels to make more nitric oxide, a fundamental molecule that helps to keep arteries soft and youthful. Of course taking a sauna will not improve muscle strength or aerobic endurance. To achieve these benefits, you will have to sweat the hard way—with a good bout of heavy exertion.

For a real boost to your health, combine sauna with a stretching exercise like yoga. Bikram yoga uses a series of yoga poses done in a studio heated to about 105 degrees Farhenheit. Hot yoga has been shown to improve strength and flexibility in addition to inducing other beneficial changes in your health, like lowering stress hormones, blood pressure, blood sugar, and improving mood and sleep. As with exercise, you need to start slowly with sauna or hot yoga, not more than ten to fifteen minutes of exposure to temperatures not more than about 120 degrees Fahrenheit at the beginning. Gradually, a tolerance to the heat develops so that most people can stay in a sauna for twenty to thirty minutes. It is not wise, however, to use temperatures above 160 to 180 degrees.

Steam baths are another popular form of heat therapy. Since most of the research has been done on sauna therapy, not steam baths, our personal intuition tells us that taking a sauna is probably somewhat more beneficial—though good hard scientific evidence comparing the two is not available.

Pregnant women should avoid the sauna. If you have a serious heart condition or other significant chronic medical issues, get clearance from your physician before starting sauna therapy. It is very important that you drink lots of water during and after a sauna. You know you are adequately hydrated if your urine is nearly clear. These disclaimers notwithstanding, studies suggest that taking a sauna is a great way to enhance overall health. We recommend adding the sauna to your fitness routine by incorporating a twenty- to thirty-minute session anywhere from once weekly to once a day. You will be amazed at the improvements in your health, appearance, mood, and sleep.

Stressed-Out? Take a Deep Breath

Whenever I feel blue, I start breathing again.
—UNKNOWN

It is becoming clear that slow, deep breathing is one of the most effective anti-stress therapies available. Dr. Andrew Weil contends that breath work may be the most important step for improving overall health and sense of well-being for many Americans. Healthy humans and other mammals show rhythmic fluctuations in heart rate and blood pressure due to the control of the autonomic nervous system. There is an ebb and flow in your body's involuntary nervous system that creates a cycle between the stress response and the relaxation response, and it occurs unconsciously every ten seconds. This yin-yang wavelike activity is influenced by your breathing, levels of activity, and arousal. In scientific studies, breathing slowly and regularly at about six times per minute has been shown to slow the heart rate, lower blood pressure, and increase calmness and well-being. Recently, the FDA approved—for the first time ever—a nondrug-based treatment for high blood pressure. If you'd like, you can spend $250 on this Resp-E-Rate monitoring device that lowers blood pressure by simply providing feedback about your breathing and coaching you to slow down your respiratory rate to about six breaths per minute. Studies show that doing this for two fifteen- to twenty-minute sessions daily will lower your blood pressure about as well as a prescription medication will.

The induction of slow and regular breathing is the common denominator of many spiritual practices, from the chants of Tibetan monks to many of the traditional prayers used by different religions around the world, such as Judaism, Islam, and Christianity. A fascinating study by Dr. Luciano Bernardi and colleagues published in the *British Medical Journal* in December 2001 found that reciting either yoga mantras or the *Ave Maria* prayer in Latin, said during the rosary slowed and regularized the breathing rate to almost exactly six cycles per minute. This study also found that chanting the prayers for six minutes or more increased the relaxation response, and improved blood flow to the brain and heart. Another study found that reciting classical poetry also slowed and regularized the breathing rate. Specifically, reading aloud Homer's *Iliad* and *Odyssey* induced a specific breathing pattern called hexameter (again, six cycles per minute), which makes it an excellent breathing exercise that is another reliable way to lower blood pressure and reduce stress hormone levels.

By synchronizing your breathing cycle with the natural waves in your autonomic activity, you amplify the relaxation response. This is an important part of the relaxing and rejuvenating effects of praying, yoga, and meditation. Slowing the breathing rate improves concentration, induces calm, reduces stress and anxiety, and, when done regularly, improves health. Dr. Bernardi suggested it may not be entirely coincidental that these different prayers all seem to slow the breath rate to about one cycle per ten seconds. The rosary was introduced to Europe by the crusaders, who learned it from the Arabs, who in turn were taught it by the Tibetan monks and the yoga masters of India. The breathing rhythm imposed by these repetitive chanting prayers or mantras induces a fixed and slowed respiration without even trying. Mantras are generally repeated about 100 times, and the rosary involves about 150 cycles. This translates to about fifteen to twenty minutes of slow deep respirations; but you can reap the same benefits whether you do it through prayer, meditation, yoga, reading classical poetry, or simply doing relaxation breathing.

Relaxation or mindful breathing requires focusing on the process of slowly and deeply inhaling and exhaling. This usually requires that you keep pulling your attention back away from the nonstop self-talk going on inside your mind and, instead, refocus on the simple act of breathing. Experts tell us that this process of refocusing activates neural pathways and, with time, can even help to strengthen your brain power the way physical exercise strengthens your body. Relaxation breathing as described below is remarkably effective at acutely lowering blood pressure by ten points or more.

Turn off the TV and try an activity such as yoga, prayer, or simply sit quietly and focus your attention on the in-and-out process of breathing for a few minutes each day. Relaxation breathing takes only a few moments, costs nothing, and can help to rebalance or de-stress your mind and body. With time and regular practice, you will notice a significant reduction in anxiety and a sense of relaxation and well-being. As an added benefit, your pulse and blood pressure may fall, and stress hormone levels may also drop.

When anxiety strikes, do some relaxation breathing exercises rather than bingeing on food. If you are struggling to fall asleep, tossing and turning in bed, shift your focus away from your worries and onto your breathing. James finds that when he is having a hard time disengaging his mind enough to fall asleep, slow deep relaxation breathing will have him drifting off into dreamland before he knows it. By the way, when you sigh it means that your brain is instinctively using a deep breath to relax your system. So when you catch yourself doing it, that may be a cue that you are feeling overstressed—a perfect time to take a few moments to do some relaxation breathing.

Relaxation Breathing

1. *Find a quiet spot. Sit in a comfortable position with your spine straight. Most people find it helpful to close their eyes.*
2. *Inhale deeply through your nose to the count of four. Relax your abdominal muscles as you breathe in. The downward movement of the diaphragm should cause your belly to protrude as your lungs fill with air.*
3. *Hold the breath for the count of seven. Keep your attention focused on your breath. If your mind wanders, bring it back to the task.*
4. *Breathe out through your mouth to the count of eight, exhaling slowly, quietly, and deeply.*
5. *Repeat this cycle at least four to eight times, which should take only a few minutes. Try to do some relaxation breathing twice per day.*

For maximal benefits, try to do 2:1 breathing; breathe in for the count of three or four and out for the count of six to eight while practicing yoga. This induces calm while also improving your strength and flexibility.

14

WHEN YOU DON'T SNOOZE, YOU LOSE

When I die, I want to go like my grandfather, who went peacefully in his sleep.
Not screaming in horror like all the passengers in his car.

—AUTHOR UNKNOWN

Sleep is a fundamental need that you may take for granted—that is, until you find yourself having trouble sleeping. We spend about one-third of our lives sleeping, and some consider it a waste of time. But we're sure you don't need us to tell you that chronic sleep deprivation makes you not just tired, but also generally irritable, unenthusiastic, unable to concentrate, and unhappy. So is sleep a waste of time? Certainly not. Life in general is just more difficult and less fun when you are sleep deprived.

It has been said that the best bridge between despair and hope is a good night's sleep. In recent years, we have learned that chronic sleep deprivation does much more than give you bloodshot eyes and a bad attitude—it can devastate your well-being by predisposing you to weight gain, diabetes, Alzheimer's disease, high blood pressure, infections, heart disease, sudden death, and stroke.

Today, we spend less time sleeping and more time snoring. Although this may be a problem that requires medical attention, there are still a variety of good options available for sleep disorders. More often, however, improving your sleep is just a matter of making a few adjustments in your lifestyle and making a good night's sleep a priority.

Throughout your waking hours, your heart is constantly struggling to respond to a variety of physical and emotional challenges that raise the level of stress hormones. These hormones (epinephrine, adrenaline, and cortisol) keep your cardiovascular system edgy and irritable. When you fall into a deep sleep, your pulse rate slows dramatically and your blood pressure falls. The blood vessels dilate, and the heart rate becomes more variable in response to the deep respirations; your cardiovascular system sighs with relief as the relaxation response kicks in.

This rest is extremely important in maintaining a healthy mind and body and healing the physiological damage that develops in response to the stresses of everyday living. When the amount or quality of your sleep is compromised, the stress hormones rise. If this becomes a chronic condition, these hormones and other disruptions in your system eventually devastate your youthful vigor and your health.

In a recent Japanese study, men who slept five hours or less per night were more than twice as likely to suffer a heart attack as men who slept eight hours nightly. Most studies addressing this question came to the conclusion that somewhere between six-and-one-half to eight hours of sleep is ideal for your overall health—especially for your heart and brain. Humans are the only species that voluntarily deprives itself of sleep. When we don't get enough of it, our bodies react as if we were under threat of an external attack. Levels of inflammation in the arteries become elevated even with relatively mild sleep deprivation. A study from Penn State University evaluated twenty-five healthy young men and women and restricted their sleep to six hours per night for one week. During the brief duration of the study, the level of cytokines (dangerous hormones that increase inflammation and predispose us to heart attack and stroke among other diseases) rose significantly. Research has also shown that C-reactive protein (CRP), a nonspecific marker of inflammation and increased cardiac risk, also becomes elevated during sleep deprivation. Thus, lack of high-quality sleep can impair your immunity and predispose you to heart attack, infections, and cancer.

Sleep Deprivation and Weight Gain

People who don't get enough sleep increase their chances of becoming overweight or obese. European investigators first noted this about a decade ago when they were puzzled to discover that the strongest predictor of childhood obesity wasn't how much television children watched but rather how long they slept each night. The less the kids slept, the heavier they tended to be. On the surface this concept seems counterintuitive; after all, we burn fewer calories while sleeping than while awake. But chronic sleep deprivation appears to disturb your hormonal profile in a manner that predisposes you to chronic hunger and overeating. Furthermore, the more overweight you become, the worse the quality of your sleep will be due to snoring and sleep apnea. So, one of the best steps you can do to stay lean and fit is to make it a priority to get seven or eight hours of sleep nightly.

A recent study at Columbia University found that people who get less than four hours of sleep were 73 percent more likely to be obese than those who got seven to nine hours. These researchers also found that the less sleep per night, the higher the risk of obesity.

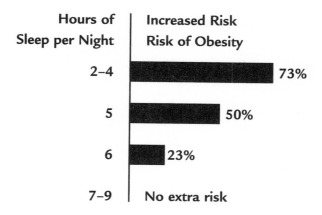

Hours of Sleep per Night	Increased Risk Risk of Obesity
2–4	73%
5	50%
6	23%
7–9	No extra risk

Source: National Health and Nutrition Examination Survey

Dr. E. Van Cauter, a sleep specialist from Chicago, studied men at baseline getting their usual seven to eight hours of nightly sleep, and then he restudied them after limiting them to only four hours of sleep per night. This trial showed that after sleep deprivation the level of leptin (a hormone that signals your brain that you're full) was inappropriately low. In other words their bodies were tricked into thinking they were low on calories, and the brain stimulated their appetites. A recent study from Stanford University looked at sleep patterns of 1,024 volunteers. The researchers documented a 15 percent increase in ghrelin (a hormone that increases hunger) and a 16 percent decrease in leptin in people who routinely slept for five hours compared with those who slept for eight. This study also showed that the less sleep an individual averaged nightly, the higher his or her weight tended to be.

Sleep deprivation increases our cortisol levels. This, in turn, stimulates the appetite and predisposes us to accumulate fat in and around the abdomen, which then increases the risk for a variety of cardiovascular problems—including diabetes and heart disease. Other studies show that sleep deprivation causes people to crave high-calorie foods such as processed carbohydrates (candy and starches), as well as salty food.

Sleep and Diabetes

Some of the most alarming data about sleep and health relates to the risk of diabetes. A recent trial reduced the amount of nightly sleep from the normal eight hours to five hours in previously healthy young adults over a period of just three days. Researchers noted a 50 percent increase in insulin resistance, which is the underlying cause of diabetes, high blood pressure, and much of the cardiovascular disease in our country.

Accelerated Aging

When laboratory animals are chronically sleep deprived, they become more susceptible to infections, lose their hair, and waste away—the equivalent of accelerating the aging process. The hormonal changes noted with disordered sleep mimic many of the changes noted with aging. For example, growth hormone is reduced even in children who are chronically low on sleep. Sleep-deprived adults also have reduced growth hormone levels, which decreases their muscle mass and increases the amount of fat, especially around the midsection. In other words, not enough sleep cranks your aging process into high gear, while seven or eight hours of restful sleep each night can slow the aging process.

Sleep Problems

America's sleep disorders can be divided into two broad categories:
- Insufficient sleep time
- Sleep apnea

The first condition can generally be remedied by simple lifestyle changes. One of the most effective methods is to reduce or eliminate caffeine. People don't realize caffeine is a long-acting stimulant that takes at least twenty-four hours to be eliminated from your system. This means that too much of it, even in the morning, can lead to tossing and turning in frustration as you struggle to fall asleep at the end of a long day. Another simple measure is to make sure you get enough physical exercise during the day to help to improve sleep quality and quantity. There is a big difference between being emotionally exhausted and physically fatigued at the end of the day. Although we are all busy from our hectic lives, if we don't exercise, we're less likely to sleep well at night. Sleep specialists also suggest a regular sleep routine whereby you go to bed and get up at about the same time every day.

As people get into their forties many find themselves awakening one or more times per night with the urge to urinate. You drag yourself out of your comfortable bed to go to the bathroom only to find that it was just a few ounces in your bladder that disrupted your rest. This nuisance problem definitely contributes to the general deterioration in sleep quality as people age. If you can "sleep like a baby" again, it will rejuvenate you by realigning your hormones to their favorable youthful state. We suggest that men begin drinking two eight-ounce glasses of soymilk daily. It should not be calcium fortified, and look for unsweetened or lightly sweetened varieties with not more than seven grams of sugar per serving—Westsoy organic unsweetened vanilla-flavored soymilk is our favorite. The phytochemical antioxidants in soy help to reduce enlargement of the prostate and minimize the spasms that cause the nighttime awakening for bathroom trips. Recent studies suggest that regular consumption of soy food may even prevent prostate cancer. In contrast, high intake of dairy products increases the problem of prostate hypertrophy and nighttime awakenings with the urge to urinate. The problem may be due to the high levels of calcium in dairy. Men who consume over two servings of dairy and more than two grams of calcium daily appear to have an increased risk of prostate cancer.

Sleep apnea is a more difficult problem. This is another common disorder, especially now that about two-thirds of Americans are overweight or obese. Sleep apnea occurs when a person's upper airway collapses during respiration while sleeping, causing loud snoring and reduced oxygenation of the body and brain. This is much more likely to occur in people as they gain weight. Losing just ten pounds can reduce the episodes of sleep apnea by 30 percent, while putting on an extra ten pounds does just the opposite.

Even though a person affected with sleep apnea appears to be sleeping eight or more hours each night, his or her heart and brain are stressed every minute or two by low oxygen levels that cause sleep disruptions. The person is then drowsy the next day, and this increases the risk of dangerous heart rhythms, such as ventricular tachycardia and sudden death. It also increases risk for diabetes, cardiovascular disease, high blood pressure, stroke, and maybe even Alzheimer's disease.

If your spouse, partner, or family member complains about your loud snoring or notices periods when you seem to stop breathing for ten to twenty seconds at a time, you probably have at least some element of sleep apnea. Weight loss is very effective for improving this condition. Milder episodes can also be treated by simply avoiding sleeping on your back. To help prevent that, you can wear a T-shirt with a pocket in the middle of the back that contains a tennis ball. This effectively prevents the sleeper from lying in the supine (faceup) position.

More serious cases of sleep apnea frequently require the use of a CPAP machine, a small device attached by a hose to a mask that provides pressurized air to your nose and mouth while you sleep. This dramatically improves the quantity and quality of sleep and has been shown to prevent cardiovascular problems—even improving the pump function of the heart.

The Instinct to Nap

Joan is the queen of napping. One of the reasons she loves having young children in the family is that it provides an excuse to nap with them each afternoon. If you, too, enjoy napping, you may be relieved to know that it is something we humans are hard-wired to do. Scientific evidence has led sleep researchers to the conclusion that nature intended us to have a midday nap. Many cultures throughout the world still incorporate a post-lunch siesta into their daily routine, especially in regions close to the equator. Even today, all around the world young children and elders take naps.

Sleep researchers have noted a universal drop in body temperature and alertness in early to midafternoon that is present even in well-rested healthy adults who are good sleepers. Experts in the field say that these changes indicate that humans are hard-wired to have a tendency to fall asleep sometime between one p.m. and four p.m., as well as at night. A heavy lunch or a poor night's sleep will accentuate this afternoon drop in vigilance and need for a nap. Studies show that even a ten-minute nap can enhance alertness, mood, and mental performance, especially after an inadequate sleep the night before. Even if you do not sleep, lying down to rest for ten to fifteen minutes in the early to midafternoon has been shown to improve mood and performance for the remainder of the day.

In our busy 24/7 world, the tradition of napping has been pushed aside in the name of productivity. This is unfortunate because a regular nap might be just the thing to rejuvenate you and improve your enjoyment of life. If you have the opportunity to take an afternoon nap, especially if you are sleep deprived for any reason, take it. You may notice a mild hangover for about five to twenty minutes while you shake off the post-nap grogginess, but once this sleep inertia dissipates, you will notice improved energy, alertness, mood, and performance. For healthy adults, naps should last ten to forty-five minutes and be avoided after four p.m.; otherwise they may disrupt your sleep quality during the night. So, if you feel like you need a nap, indulge yourself and don't feel guilty. Science tells us it is a natural, relaxing means to help you achieve your optimum performance.

Steps to Improve Your Sleep and Rejuvenate Your Life

1. *Exercise daily and maintain a healthy weight. Aerobic and weight training are both important. The more energy you expend while you are awake, the better you will sleep at night. Try to add some yoga or Pilates to your routine because they are great for inducing relaxation and improving sleep quality.*

2. *If you drink caffeine, do it before lunchtime and avoid it for the remainder of the day. Avoid other stimulants altogether.*

3. *Make sure your bedroom is quiet, very dark, and cool, and your bed is comfortable.*

4. *Reserve the bed for sleep and sex.*

5. *For men, drink two glasses of unsweetened non–calcium fortified soymilk daily to prevent nighttime bathroom trips.*

6. *Consider taking a hot bath or shower shortly before bedtime. A twenty- to thirty-minute hot sauna is even better to set you up for a great night's sleep.*

7. *Don't drink fluids after dinner, and no alcohol starting four hours before bedtime. Avoid large meals late in the evening.*

8. *Develop a quiet bedtime ritual to calm your mind and prepare you to fall asleep. Try reading quietly, listening to calming music, relaxation breathing, praying, or yoga.*

9. *Effective, safe prescription sleeping meds are an option that is best reserved for unusual circumstances where temporary sleep disturbances are to be expected, such as a trip across several time zones. Nearly all prescription sleeping pills can be habit-forming if used regularly. Aspirin is a surprisingly effective agent for inducing sleep. We've found that even 81 mg can be effective in this role. Do not use more than a 325 mg dose, and never take aspirin on an empty stomach, since it can cause stomach ulcers and serious bleeding.*

10. *Establish a consistent routine about what time you go to bed and when you arise. Try to maintain the same sleep schedule seven nights per week; don't try to catch up by sleeping in late on Saturday and Sunday.*

11. *Don't obsess about insomnia that occurs infrequently. Relax and realize that occasional difficulty in sleeping is just an inconvenience, not a serious health problem. If you find yourself having a hard time falling asleep, try the relaxation breathing described in the previous chapter.*

12. *Try to avoid very strenuous exercise within a couple hours of going to bed.*

15

HURRY, SCURRY, WORK, AND WORRY

Most people have overestimated how much money they need,
and have miscalculated the work-to-play ratio . . . Except us.

—TOM AND RAY MAGLIOZZI, ON *CAR TALK*

The "French Paradox" is the phenomenon whereby the people of France have very low rates of heart disease in spite of the fact that they eat a higher fat diet and smoke more cigarettes than Americans. This cardioprotection has been attributed to their love affair with red wine, but we suspect the French Paradox is more likely to be a benefit of their relaxed pace of life. The French call it their "joie de vivre," or joy of life.

Over the past two decades, the French have shortened their workweek to thirty-five hours while, at the same time, we Americans now toil fifty-four hours per week. They enjoy leisurely social dinners lasting until late evening; we gulp our meals at fast-food restaurants as we hurry between commitments. They say we Americans live to work, while the French work only so they can live.

Our lives are too short to live them just for work. As important as you think you are on the job, if you died tomorrow, you would be replaced in a few weeks' time. Although you might hate to admit it, life at your workplace would carry on just fine without you. On the other hand, your family and friends would be devastated if you suddenly disappeared. Their world would be disrupted permanently, and they would miss you for the rest of their lives. It is easy to fall into the trap of believing that earning a living is our top priority in life. But our main concerns should be enjoying life, caring for ourselves and the people we love, and spending our free time pursuing our passions instead of accumulating "stuff."

The American motto may be "more is better," but as far as your heart is concerned, less is more. We spend more time at work than anyone else in the industrialized world. Incredibly, medieval peasants even worked fewer hours than the average American today. Many of our nonworking hours are spent shopping; we spend money we don't have and buy things we don't need to impress people who don't care. Then we end up with a lot of stuff that burns up our little remaining free time and energy. Our land of plenty has turned into a nation of excess. John de Graaf has led a nationwide "Take Back Your Time" movement. One of its mottos is "More Time. Less Stuff," because Americans are number one in the world when it comes to stuff per capita. De Graaf argues that we would all be happier if we traded some of the productivity gains in America for more time instead of more money and more things. We agree that what we need most for our health and happiness is a little less of everything—less work, less stress, less shopping, less stuff, and definitely less calories.

Your heart thrives on simplicity. We are not hard-wired for the fast pace of modern life. Remember when you were a kid and it seemed like there was never enough time to do all the nothing you wanted to do? When we are chronically trying to do too many things at the same time, we are left feeling constantly as though we are running behind and need to pick up the pace. This harried lifestyle takes a toll on our health and well-being. As Lily Tomlin said, "The trouble with the rat race is that even if you win, you're still a rat."

A constant sense of time urgency activates our "fight or flight" system. This elevates blood pressure and heart rate and stresses our cardiovascular system and can lead to hypertension, depression, and ultimately even heart attack and stroke. Life is short; and paradoxically, the faster we rush, the more quickly our precious time evaporates. The journey is the destination. The time to enjoy life is right now, right here.

Day in and day out many of the patients we see are suffering from anxiety, sleep problems, chronic pain, high blood pressure, obesity, and depression. Taking proper care of yourself takes time, and this is a vanishing resource in our lives today. Dr. Suzanne Schweikert writes, "An hour a day could keep the doctor away." The latest recommendations emphasize that an hour of exercise daily is optimal for health, but with

Americans working an entire month more each year than they did thirty-five years ago, few of us seem to find the time for physical activity. James asks his overworked, over-booked, overstressed, and overweight patients, "What fits into your busy schedule better, an hour of exercise each day or being debilitated or dead twenty-four hours a day?"

So what's a frenetic, multitasking, workaholic American to do? Get your rest and take your vacations. Learn to say no more often. When you try to do everything all the time, you end up doing nothing well, and eventually, your whole existence can start to feel like a burden. At least twice a day, try to turn off all the noise of the busy world, including the radio and TV—just clear your mind. Do not get in the habit of working late or bringing work home with you each evening. Instead, reserve long workdays and homework for urgent deadlines. Don't feel guilty about just kicking back sometimes; relaxation is neither frivolous nor self-indulgent. Your mental sharpness, emotional resilience, health, and productivity improve if you frequently make it a point to unwind. Treat yourself regularly to a vacation where you have the chance to relax, day-dream, and enjoy the natural beauty around you, rather than rushing from one spot to the next. Try to protect your days off and don't overbook them with errands and other busywork. Make it a priority to take pleasure in preparing and eating nourishing meals at home and boycott the processed fast-food routine. Life moves pretty quickly. If you don't stop and have some fun once in a while, you could miss it.

Mindfulness: Reawaken Your Senses

Because of all this unhealthy rushing around, mindfulness has become a hot topic today. Becoming more mindful requires staying in the moment, slowing down, and realizing that our entire lives happen in the here and now. Think back over the decades of your life and make a note of the memories that stand out. We can still see the cloud-swept sky and feel the cool autumn breeze near the small lake where we used to live twenty years ago. It seems strange that often we are left with vivid mental snapshots of seemingly ordinary occurrences. The common denominator of the memories that are more likely to become crystallized forever in your consciousness is that they are moments when you are fully engaged in the here and now, experiencing it with all your senses.

The goal of mindfulness meditation is to tune in rather than zone out. Mindfulness training can be helpful for improving stress or treating chronic illnesses like depression, obesity, and high blood pressure. One of the simplest and easiest ways to become more mindful is to take a few minutes in a quiet environment to just focus on breathing slowly and deeply. Or go outside and take a walk, and just clear your mind as you concentrate on walking and breathing and the natural environment around you. At mealtime, try to eat slowly and chew your food thoroughly while focusing on the taste and texture of the food rather than absentmindedly gulping it down. When you slow down to enjoy the food, you will be less likely to overeat.

Despite what the mass media would have us believe, we are much more than our job, our possessions, and our net worth; and prizes are not awarded to the person who dies with the most things. Our time, energy, and love of the people in our lives are what we value most, and our heart knows this instinctively and responds wonderfully well to less stress and more relaxation.

To be honest, this chronic time urgency is a problem we struggle with on a daily basis. When we took our family to the Mediterranean coast of France last summer, we found their more relaxed pace of life like a breath of fresh air.

> You only live once, but if you work it right, once is enough.
> —JOE E. LEWIS

Steps to a Simpler, More Enjoyable Life

1. *Just say no.* Do only the things you need and you want to do; make sure you have plenty of white space left on your calendar. Time you enjoyed wasting was not a waste of time. When you feel stressed or overbooked, ask yourself, "Will this matter five years from now?" If the answer is no, *blow it off.* Sometimes more than anything else you just need a little personal time to decompress and regroup. Learn to set limits and don't be afraid to say no. And don't feel guilty about it—you can't do it all.

2. *Make your sleep a priority.* Get seven to eight hours of sleep nightly. Take a short afternoon nap, if you need it. Farmers let fields lie fallow for a year to revitalize the soil. Elite athletes ease off the intensity of their workouts before a major competition to ensure a peak performance. Rest and relaxation are keys to optimal health.

3. *Eat meals with your family and friends.* Take your time, turn off the TV and computer. Have a glass of wine, relax, chat, and enjoy the food and the company.

4. *When you feel stressed, take a deep breath.* Find a quiet spot and just focus on your breathing.

5. *Count your blessings.* Quit worrying—it is a misuse of imagination and a worthless waste of time and energy. Stop moping about the past and pining about the future. Live in the moment. Today is a gift; perhaps that's why it is called "the present." Simple pleasures are the best—if you want to feel rich, just count all the blessings you have that money cannot buy. An attitude of gratitude is a surefire way to stay young and improve your health and happiness. When you find yourself bogged down in one of those days that seem to hold just one discouragement after another, think about all the blessings that you have. Not your new car or your financial assets, but the blessings that really matter like the love of your family, spouse, and friends, your health, and the fact that you are alive. Focus on the positive aspects of your life, all those things that only you can truly appreciate. This may not make the worries, disappointments, and struggles of your life disappear, but optimism and gratitude will help you find the inner strength to cope with life's problems in a healthy, productive way.

6. *Out you go.* Stay connected to the natural world—it has the power to clear your mind and nurture your soul. At the warp speed of modern life, we usually don't even notice the roses, let alone stop to smell them. We are part of the web of life, so let the rhythms of nature soothe your harried heart. Watch the clouds sail overhead, gaze into the twinkling night sky, watch the dancing flames in a fireplace, or listen to the crashing waves on the shore. The sights, sounds, smells, and feel of our native milieu have a remarkable calming effect on your heart and mind. Nature provides a silent stillness and beauty that resonates with our instincts, refreshing and relaxing us. *Our time here is short, and now is our moment in the sun—don't miss it.*

7. *Tune out the static.* Studies show that chronic noise increases cortisol (a steroid stress hormone), especially when it's in the form of the TV and radio blaring messages mostly about violence and other disturbing problems. It is difficult to be happy and relaxed when you are constantly barraged by upsetting images and noise. A quiet spot to sleep at night is important for your health. The channels in your brain that monitor auditory stimuli are always open, even while you

are sleeping, and noises, not loud enough to wake you up have been shown to increase your level of cortisol the next day. So lose the cuckoo clock, turn off the TV, and take breaks from watching the news. If you have a raucous neighborhood use a white-noise recording that makes it sound as if you were sleeping in a quiet ocean-side bungalow.

8. *Grow up without growing old.* We do not stop playing because we get too old. We become old because we quit playing. Staying young comes naturally when you maintain an adventurous, curious, open-minded attitude and a fun, active lifestyle. Give yourself permission to be playful again and make enjoying time with your friends a priority. Do things that make you feel young again. If you have forgotten how, just hang around young people, and it will all come back to you.

9. *When you ain't got nothin', you got nothin' to lose.* Can you recall the time when you first left home and everything you owned fit into the trunk of a small car? An unfettered life engenders a real sense of freedom. To the extent that your possessions possess you, they are a curse. By the time you pay for, clean, organize, worry about, and insure all your stuff, you end up spending your free time as a maintenance person. What you pay attention to will thrive. Therefore, invest your energy in maintaining your body and your personal relationships. You will have more time and more fun!

10. *Don't take life so seriously; it's not permanent.* Learn to laugh at yourself. When you make fun of others, you often alienate people. When you make fun of yourself, you make friends. If you lose your ability to laugh, you will have a hard time coping and keeping life in the perspective. Perhaps the biggest waste of all is a day without laughter and joy.

Chronic Emotional Stress Might Be Making You Fat

Donald is one of our patients, a delightful fifty-nine-year-old who struggles with high blood pressure, sleep apnea, and obesity around his midsection. Lately he has been under increased stress related to work demands, and his weight problem has worsened. He admits that he often finds himself shuffling out to the kitchen in the middle of the night to compulsively raid the pantry. During one of these sessions, he will often wolf down one or two packages of Hostess Snowballs before he even realizes what he doing. Scientific evidence indicates that this "night-eating syndrome" is linked to elevated stress hormones.

Studies consistently show that both humans and animals who live in high-stress environments tend to put on belly fat–the unhealthy adipose tissue that accumulates in and around the intra-abdominal organs. A report that appeared in the July 2005 medical journal *Brain, Behavior, and Immunity* studied the connection between stress and food choices. This study found that rats, when subjected to stressful living conditions, chose unhealthy foods like sugar water more often. Emotional distress in both people and animals raises stress hormones, including cortisol, which compels them to crave comfort or junk foods such as sweet, salty, and fatty treats.

The problem of an expanding waistline can create a vicious cycle. Living with chronic stress elevates cortisol and other hormones that cause storage of excess fat around the midsection. This increased belly fat in turn appears to exaggerate the body's response to stress (see below). A Yale University study published in the fall of 2004 compared overweight women of differing shapes and found that those with the larger waists (apple-shaped) secreted more cortisol when subjected to stress than the women with big hips, but relatively small waists (pear-shaped).

STRESS AND BELLY FAT: THE VICIOUS CYCLE

Chronic Stress

Sleep Apnea,
High BP, Diabetes, etc.

Increased
Cortisol Levels

Worsening Obesity

Cravings for Junk
Foods and Sweets

More Cravings
for Junk Foods

Increased Fat
in Abdomen

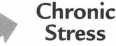

Further Increase in Cortisol and
Exaggerated Responses to Stress

Excessive visceral (belly) fat is not just a cosmetic issue, but also a serious health problem. Minimizing the stress in your life will not just make you happier, it can also make you healthier and more attractive. Most people trying to lose weight do not understand the importance of this stress-obesity connection. If you want to become lean and fit again, it helps to get your stress levels down. Exercise, including gentler activities such as yoga and walking, will not only burn calories, but also may change the way your body responds to stress. Other effective stress-relieving endeavors include meditation, prayer, vacations, and prioritizing your life so as to spend more leisure time enjoying your family and friends.

The Deadly Rush Hour

> Have you ever noticed that anyone driving slower than you is an idiot,
> and anyone driving faster than you is a maniac?
> —GEORGE CARLIN

There is something about driving in rush-hour city traffic that tends to bring out hostility even in otherwise mild-mannered people. A new survey showed that 54 percent of Americans experience stress during their daily commute. It's not surprising that heavy traffic and longer commute times were major predictors of whether or not the commuter felt stressed. Other aggravating issues included running late, bad weather, detours, delays, air/noise pollution, and hostile fellow commuters. Mondays seemed to be the worst day, which coincides with the day of the week that is most deadly for heart attacks, sudden death, and stroke.

A study published in the *New England Journal of Medicine* in October 2004 found that heart attack patients were three times more likely to have been driving or riding in traffic the hour before their attack. And it wasn't just the automobile drivers, bus passengers, and bicyclists were also noted to suffer heart attacks more often after riding in heavy traffic. According to the researchers, the increased risk appeared to be more a function of smoggy conditions than noise or stress. Many other scientific papers have documented the increased heart risk posed by air pollution, especially the particles belched out by diesel engines. Smog causes inflammation in the blood vessels that can sometimes lead to rupture of plaques resulting in a heart attack. It also disrupts the heart's natural rhythms, increases stress hormones, and constricts blood vessels.

Research shows that air pollution can be a surprisingly localized risk. For example, people riding in cars or buses inhale ten times more pollutants and toxic compounds than folks in the same vicinity who are walking on the sidewalk, where the tailpipe emissions are not pointed directly at them. The take-home message is to avoid smoggy conditions whenever possible. Try to use less congested routes and travel at nonpeak times when and if you can. When exercising, stay away from busy streets and look for less-traveled roads and parks. The pollution at airports is generally among the worst in the city, so try to avoid spending unnecessary time there.

Is there a solution to getting stressed-out behind the wheel? Remember that getting mad at other drivers does no one any good, especially you—road rage takes a toll on your heart and diminishes your sense of well-being. Chill out and listen to music, a favorite radio program, or a book on tape. Take advantage of the windshield time by doing some relaxation breathing. Think of driving as an opportunity to relax, instead of a frustration that leaves you even more tightly wound. Joan often says that once we are in the car and on our way to a destination, we should not think about making up time; "When we get there, we get there," is her attitude. It is the sense of time urgency that can make driving unpleasant—and more dangerous.

Too Noisy to Hear Yourself Think

James often awakes early and goes for a three-mile run with our two border collies. As the sun rises the only sounds he hears are the chirping of birds and the wind in the trees. Under a sky changing from black to blue, the clouds drift overhead, and he can breathe fresh clean air. Moments like these rejuvenate the mind, invigorate the body, and make us happy to be alive. Silent stillness can bring energy, inspiration, and strength, just as excessive noise can drain your vital force and creativity.

Sometimes we need to seek out refuge from the clatter of modern life. Some people have become so used to noise that they feel uncomfortable with silence. You probably know that too much noise can leave you stone deaf or get you arrested for disturbing the peace, but you might be surprised to learn that chronic high-level noise exposure can also predispose you to a heart attack. This was the conclusion of a recent study of over 4,000 German patients that evaluated the effects of ever-present irritating noise from industrial plants, construction work, automobile and truck traffic, etc., on the risk of myocardial infarction. The results were based on the estimated accumulated exposure to noxious noise over a ten-year period preceding a heart attack. Interestingly, the study showed that women exposed to high levels of environmental noise were 50 percent more likely to suffer a heart attack than the women who did not have to endure a deafening clamor on a daily basis. Even men, the less sensitive gender, still showed a 30 percent increased risk of heart attack when having to live and/or work in a noisy environment.

Multiple studies have documented that chronic high-level exposure to irritating sounds increases blood pressure and elevates stress hormones. We are learning that these disturbances in the autonomic nervous system play an important role in long-term risk of heart disease. We don't know how much noise it takes to increase cardiovascular risk, but the threshold is likely to differ from one person to the next. Joan, who grew up as a solitary child in a tranquil home, is especially sensitive to excessive noise and commotion. Her parents were forty-six and forty-eight years old when she was born. Even her extended family is tiny—we joke that she could have her family reunion in the bathroom of a room at the Holiday Inn. Yet today she lives in a household with four active, noisy children and three dogs who howl at anything that moves. Even the three cats occasionally awaken us in the middle of the night when they hawk hairballs on our bedroom rug. TVs blare and music rattles the windowpanes while the doorbells, phones, fax, and beeper ring incessantly. Joan sometimes complains, "I can't hear myself think in all this noise and commotion."

Serenity and silence, like wilderness and wildlife, are concepts that grow dearer as they vanish to the point of extinction. Humans developed as a species in a milieu of relative calm. The soothing voices of nature in the form of singing birds and whispering winds provided most of the background sound until the relatively recent blossoming of the highly mechanized modern world. Dr. Gregg Jacobs believes "the hyperstimulation of the modern world threatens our health and well-being by depriving us of the calm and tranquility that is our evolutionary birthright." Silence and solitude are essential elements of our life, and just like water or omega-3 fats, if we do not get our minimum requirement of them on a regular basis, it is difficult to stay physically and emotionally healthy.

Silence and solitude provide the fertile soil that spawns ideas, insights, and inspiration. The greatest discoveries in science and masterpieces of art were generally inspired by moments of silent reflection. A quiet, calm environment allows the mind to wander and enhances imagination and problem solving. Occasional solitude can improve our ability to cope with stress, and can also be a wellspring of self-discovery, spirituality, and ingenuity. Numbed by noise and distracted by multi-tasking, many people have lost touch with their inner self. We have become addicted to a barrage of meaningless banter and insignificant images all mostly irrelevant, forgettable, and disposable.

Even a few minutes of peace can be uplifting in certain settings. Sometimes an hour or two after putting the kids to bed, we steal upstairs to make sure they are comfortable and safe. To us, there is nothing more heartwarming and reassuring than the sight of Kathleen, Caroline, and Evan peacefully sleeping. They breathe deeply and softly as they dream of their world that is unfolding before them. As we gently tuck in their blankets and their kiss them on the cheek, everything seems right with the world, if only for those few peaceful moments.

16

LOVE, HOSTILITY, AND SURVIVAL

The best and most beautiful things in the world cannot be seen or even touched.
They must be felt with the heart.

—HELEN KELLER

Over time, people have come to the same puzzling conclusion that love and many other emotions originate in the heart, just as they correctly assumed that intellect comes from the brain. Why did this idea about the relationship of love and the heart emerge and why, if this is just an old wives' tale, is the notion so pervasive from culture to culture? The heart, a tireless workhorse that powers and nurtures every cell in your body, is essentially only a bag of muscle—a durable and efficient blood pump. So what's love go to do with it?

The mind-body connection exerts a powerful influence on our health, and nowhere is this more evident than in the cardiovascular system. Emotions like love and hate may not emanate from the heart, but they are transmitted from the brain to the cardiovascular system almost instantaneously, resulting in minute-to-minute fluctuations in blood pressure and pulse and exerting profound long-term influences on cardiovascular health and even overall survival. Caring about others and feeling cared about does not just bring meaning to life, it can actually help to keep you alive and vigorous.

The connection between emotions and the heart is not difficult to perceive. When you enjoy the company of someone you love or help someone in need, when you hold a precious baby or grandchild or pet your dog—you have a physical response. Your blood vessels dilate and your heart relaxes and slows its pace. If you take notice, you can feel a sense of calm and well-being radiating through your cardiovascular system.

Anything that promotes connection to a community or a sense of love or altruism improves health and healing, especially in the cardiovascular system. On the other hand, when you are in conflict, expressing anger, hate or fear, or harshly criticizing others, your blood vessels constrict, your heart pounds, your blood pressure shoots up, and many people, even those with normal hearts, report a sense of tightness in the chest. Chronic negative emotions and stress can lead to heart disease and illness. Stress has been shown to play a major role in the development of up to 80 percent of medical disorders. Essentially, anything that results in a sense of isolation or antagonism can lead to sickness and premature death. An analysis of the NHLBI Family Heart Study published in *Archives of Internal Medicine* in December 2004 found that hostility increased blood sugar, inflammation, blood pressure, and triglycerides and lowered the good HDL cholesterol. These changes all worsen the risk of heart disease, stroke, diabetes, and Alzheimer's disease, and they age you before your time.

To Love and Be Loved Brings You Courage and Strength

We live in a superconnected global village. We can communicate faster, farther, and easier than ever before with the simple touch of a keyboard or a cell phone. In reality, however, our interpersonal network, the fabric of social support, has been unraveling. Scattered extended families, frequent job changes and relocations, and the weakening of family, community, and neighborhood ties have all left us increasingly lonely for meaningful human relationships.

Ironically, in the age of communication and connections, we are even more isolated, and this can lead to distrust, suspicion, loneliness, and hostility. These feelings can close us off emotionally, exposing us to disease and aging, especially of the heart and blood vessels. Life at times is difficult, and a single individual, like a single thread, can be easily broken when placed under stress. But when woven into a fabric of tight social support, that person becomes exponentially stronger and more resilient to the stresses of life. American men in particular are born and raised to be independent mavericks. The price they pay is a life expectancy that is six years shorter than our more socially connected wives, mothers, daughters, and sisters.

Love and connectedness will sustain you to withstand the ravages of time and stress. Your ability to thrive is dependent upon the healing powers of positive relationships, and quality is more important than quantity when it comes to the influence of these ties on your long-term health and vitality. Even the presence of just one close confidant has been shown to provide strong health and emotional benefits.

A lone warrior operating in constant *fight or flight* mode may win a few battles, but he won't survive a lifelong war. Many women instinctively respond to stress by nurturing and forging alliances rather than through aggression or escape. This is referred to as a *"tend and befriend"* reaction to stress, and is a much more effective tool for long-term survival strategy in our modern world.

Both nurturing and being nurtured provide soothing and healing effects, especially to the cardiovascular system, in ways that we are only beginning to understand. Generally, physicians avoid using the "L" word perhaps because it sounds unprofessional or unscientific. Intimacy, nurturing, interpersonal connections, community, and social support are synonyms for LOVE in the language of "medicalese." Although research consistently shows the presence or absence of love to be among the most powerful risk factors for heart disease, the topic continues to be largely ignored by mainstream medicine.

The relationship between social isolation and cardiovascular disease and death has been examined in at least eight separate large community-based studies over the past two decades. Theses studies involved communities ranging from Sweden and Finland to California. They involved tens of thousands of people, and they all came to the same consistent conclusions: People who were socially isolated experienced a three- to fivefold increased risk of premature death from all causes compared to those who have a strong sense of connection and community.

One of these studies, "The Beta-Blocker Heart Attack Trial," evaluated 2,300 men who survived a heart attack. Those who were socially isolated and emotionally stressed had four times the risk of death, even after controlling for genetics, smoking, diet, exercise, and weight. Good social support conferred much more powerful benefits than did the beta-blocker medication, even though the message physicians took away from that trial was that beta-blockers improved survival after heart attack.

Women who are in happy marriages are healthier than unmarried women. However, a woman in an unhappy marriage has no health advantage. Married men on the other hand seem to be healthier than unmarried men regardless of whether or not they report that they are happily married. In May 2005, Eric Loucks, PhD, reported a study showing that men with stronger social networks had lower levels of inflammation in their systems. Social connections such as being married, having friends and relatives in whom they can confide, and involvement in religious or community organizations appear to prevent inflammation and its attendant dangers like heart disease and cancer.

Dean Ornish, MD, in his excellent book *Love and Survival*, confides something that we have long suspected to be true: The major benefits of his intensive lifestyle-altering programs are at least in part due to the extensive social support his patients receive in daily group sessions—more so than even the diet and exercise components of the program.

It has been said that of all the things in our lives, it would be most difficult to live without love (but toilet paper comes in a close second). Love and intimacy are at the core of both what causes and what heals illness. If a new drug was discovered that had the healing and longevity powers that love has, virtually every physician in the country would embrace it for use on all of their patients. Unfortunately, we doctors are not taught much about the curative power of love and intimacy in medical school. Instead, modern medicine generally focuses on pharmaceutical agents and high-tech devices, chemicals and molecules, microorganisms, and surgeries. Still, no single factor in human biology—not diet, not tobacco, not physical activity, not genes, not drugs, not weight, not surgeries—has a more profound effect on our chances of staying healthy, happy, and alive than a sense of connectedness. Its loss can adversely impact our health in many different ways.

Here are some suggestions for improving your health and longevity by focusing on strength from relationships:

- Invest more time and energy in friends and family.
- Work on communicating more openly.
- Find group support. Surround yourself with a community.

- Be quick to forgive and forget. It has been said that the key to happiness is good health and a short memory.
- Commit yourself to a noble cause that you care about. Try to include altruism and service in your life.
- Engage the therapeutic effect of touch.
- Develop more compassion and empathy for both yourself and others.
- Appreciate the interconnectedness of all life on Earth.

All Life Is One

In order to have the motivation to follow through on all of this book's recommendations about diet, exercise, and lifestyle, you need to be inspired, have a strong sense of purpose in life, and possess high self-esteem. Finding your purpose nearly always involves making a positive impact on the life around us.

You probably think of yourself as an independent being, fully capable of supporting yourself. The truth is that you are not much different from one of the single cells among the trillions of cells that make up your body. You came into this world as an extension of your mother and father, and survived only because of the love and attention of those who nurtured you. The life-sustaining oxygen in every breath you take is present only as a by-product of the plants of the earth—without our green friends there would be no humans or any other animals on this planet. Every calorie you consume can be ultimately traced back to another life-form since all life on Earth is one. When you awaken to this reality, the road back to health, happiness, and fitness becomes easier to find and follow.

Life is generally intolerant of living entities that are not remaining true to their nature and working toward the good of the whole. At a very fundamental level, life is about sustaining life in the future. Humans are among the most socially interdependent of all the animals, and we must remain true to our genetic identity if we are to stay vigorous, fit, and fulfilled. In other words, the best way to be happy is to make others so. A selfish and self-absorbed human becomes miserable and unhealthy both mentally and physically.

To be happy and healthy, we need someone and/or something to love, something to do, and something to look forward to with enthusiasm. Virtually every weight-loss program you will try is doomed to fail unless the emotional element of self-respect is in place. Until you appreciate your inner self, it is difficult to improve your outer self. In order to make positive and permanent changes, you will need to learn to respect yourself. If you make a positive difference, however small, in the community of life around you, you will begin to feel the energy and enthusiasm flow back into your existence. Happy and healthy go hand in hand. The converse is also true: Cranky people generally do not feel well. Self-centeredness can create a vicious downward spiral created by obsessing on your worries or pain as you grow weaker and sicker and more self-absorbed. It is hard to be happy if you feel weak, sickly, or in pain. Joan is always reminding the children, and James, "It's not all about you." A life full of love, health, and happiness grows out of an attitude of caring and generosity.

Love is not meant purely in the traditional romantic sense, but encompasses anything that engages you in a constructive, cooperative process. In the Tecumseh Community Health Study, 3,000 men and women were studied for approximately ten years. After adjustments for the usual risk factors, men reporting the highest levels of social relationships and activities lived the longest. The most protective of the various activities were those that involved regular volunteer work. Those who volunteered to help others at least once a week were two and one-half times less likely to die than those who never volunteered. In other words, those who helped others lived longer themselves. Donating blood on a regular basis is an example of volunteerism that has been shown in several scientific studies to be good for your health.

Do you enjoy gardening? Studies show that regular gardening provides as much protection against sudden cardiac death as regular aerobic walking or running. Nurturing plants is a good form of exercise, and it also connects you to other living things. Gardening brings many people outside of their self-absorbed ruminations, doubts, and worries. It provides an opportunity to show love, because you are doing something that "your heart is in." Even work can be good for your heart if it is a "labor of love." Find a job or even a hobby that allows you to use your talents to make a positive difference in your world.

Why do intimacy and connectedness seem to help the heart? Although an unexplored frontier, it is self-evident that when we share our problems, we ease the burden of stress on your system. It is as though sharing your life with loved ones and friends halves your sorrows and doubles your joys. Connecting with the web of life around you lowers the levels of stress hormones like adrenaline and cortisol, and increases activity in the parasympathetic nervous system. This soothes the irritated, overreactive cardiovascular system typical of a hostile, frightened, or isolated person, and decreases the risks of heart attack, stroke, and death. In the final analysis, it comes down to a pretty simple concept: Being a good-hearted person will leave you with a healthy heart.

Waste Not, Want Not: the Cycle (and Recycle) of Life

I grew up in the sixties with practical parents who were children of the Great Depression. My father was the king of recycling before they had a name for it, when it was simply considered being thrifty. Having his old shoes resoled and reconditioned made Dad happier than a buying a pair of new shoes. For more than forty years, rather than waste gasoline driving each day, he walked the three-mile round-trip to and from work. He never threw a returnable can or bottle in the garbage, nor would he walk past one on the road without stopping to pick it up.

My mother, who today remains as down-to-earth and practical as ever, scrubbed aluminum foil clean after cooking on it so she could use it again. Cotton diapers were washed and used time after time, growing softer for the wear. Their marriage was strong, their dreams focused, and their values rock solid. I can picture them now: Dad in Bermuda shorts, T-shirt, and a Minnesota Twins baseball hat; Mom in a housedress, baby in one arm, and dish towel in other.

It was an age during which broken things were fixed rather than trashed. The black-and-white television, the screen door, the hand-me-down clothes with patches over the knees and elbows—stuff was made almost good as new, not just discarded and replaced. A single bathtub of water could get six children squeaky clean; even if the water going down the drain was pretty dirty by the time the last kid climbed out of the tub. "Waste not, want not" was the motto of a generation who had lived through times of scarcity and felt the quiet desperation of sometimes wanting for needs as basic as food and shelter. Their frugal ways at times drove me crazy—all that mending, reusing, sharing, and conserving—sometimes I just longed for the luxury of being wasteful. Waste implied prosperity, being able to discard things meant you were confident there would always be more.

Then my father died, and on that cold January night, I was hit with the anguish of understanding that sometimes there isn't any more. Sometimes, the possessions we care about most become used up and disappear . . . never to return. So we need to love and care for the people and things in our world. Support them when they are weak, mend relationships when they are broken, heal wounds that still fester, and safeguard our blessings. Conserve and cherish them, hold them close to our hearts. This is the case for sometimes rocky marriages and old cars, for kids with dreadful report cards, dogs with weak bladders and bad hips, and aging parents and grandparents. We keep them because they are worth it, and because they make our lives worth living. Our planet too needs our love, respect, and nurturing. We are given the privilege of living in this paradise for one short lifetime. Yet the future of our children's children and the earth itself depends upon us preserving our world so that we leave it as good as we found it when we inherited it from our ancestors.

The most important things in life can't be replaced: the beauty and harmony of nature, a parent or a sibling, a child or a grandparent, or a special pet, or a friend and classmate that might be half a continent away. These things bring meaning and pleasure to our lives; they make our existence precious. So we try to stay close even when we are separated by hundreds or thousands of miles. Family and good friends are kind of like the stars in the sky—although you can't always see them, they are always out there, shining in the darkness, helping us navigate the world, bringing warmth and light to our lives.

Your Pet: A Best Friend to Keep You Young and Healthy

You can say any foolish thing to a dog, and the dog will give you a look that says,
"My God, you're right! I never would've thought of that!"
—DAVE BARRY

Many Americans today feel isolated, lonely, and depressed, which only aggravates problems like obesity and heart disease. James sometimes sends folks like these home with a formal signed prescription that reads, "One dog or cat to be taken for a walk or hugged twice daily." Our family can vouch for the fact that nothing brightens up a day better than the enthusiastic unconditional love, loyalty, and companionship of a good pet (or three).

A study published in the March 2003 issue of the *American Journal of Cardiology* by Dr. Erica Friedmann showed that heart patients who owned a pet experienced less anxiety, depression, and anger following a heart attack. Another study in that journal showed that about 7 percent of people who did not own a pet died during the first year following a heart attack, compared to only 1 percent of those who did own a pet. This benefit seemed to be strongest for dog owners, but was also present to a lesser degree for owners of other animals.

Nurturing another living creature brings us outside of our own worries, and is a powerful source of happiness and healing. Petting a dog or cat lowers blood pressure, and older people show improved overall health, self-esteem, and mood, resulting in decreased health-care utilization when caring for a dog or a cat. Pets seem to somehow shelter their owners from stress-related illnesses like heart disease and hypertension. The blood levels of dangerous hormones like cortisol and norepinephrine are much lower during stress when a pet dog or cat is by its owner's side than when the person is alone or even when the person's spouse is next to him or her.

H. Jackson Brown writes: "Hold puppies, kittens, and babies every chance you get." Joan has always said she can just feel the beneficial hormones like oxytocin coursing through her system when she cuddles with a newborn baby. A study by Rebecca Johnson, a professor at the University of Missouri Veterinary School, found that affectionately or playfully interacting with a dog increased people's levels of the "feel-good" hormones—serotonin, prolactin, and oxytocin. Think of petting a friendly dog and getting dog kisses in the form of licks is a great way to realign your hormonal profile to a healthy and happy state.

Keep the Fires of Passion Burning

It's not just a coincidence that scalding hot water burns and an affectionate hug feels nice. We come hard-wired with these and countless other mammalian instincts to help us navigate the often perilous waters of life. The strongest instinct is the compelling impulse to procreate, and it evolved to ensure the survival of the species.

"Nature intended for sex to be pleasurable; an exquisite reproductive itch," as author Jeffrey Kluger of *Time* magazine writes. The yearning to scratch that itch is a powerful force that shapes human behavior. J. Gayle Beck, professor of psychology at the University of Buffalo, puts it this way: "All creatures do things that feel good and avoid things that feel bad. The individuals who learn that best live longest."

However, the power of human touch extends far beyond sexuality. There is loving reassurance in a mother's caress for her child. Even fifty years after the fires of lust first drew them together, simple hand-holding or a hug can bring a couple the same sense of affection and unity. Physical contact—the warm, soft touch of skin to skin—can soothe our anxieties, and strengthen our immunity, and save lives. Like all mammals, humans thrive when they are loved and nurtured and wither when they are isolated and lonely. An infamous study from the early 1900s set out to prove the newly advanced germ theory by minimizing person-to-person contact and thereby preventing infections in newborns in orphanages. The babies in these institutions were placed in strict isolation and were never picked up or touched unless absolutely necessary. The study, published in 1915, reported that among ten institutions using this practice, not a single baby under age two survived. Affection and loving touch are among the most essential nutrients to our physical and emotional well-being.

One of the simplest and most powerful predictors of long-term health among married people is the response to the question: Does your spouse show you his or her love? If the answer is no, it's a problem that is worth some attention. By the way, the surest way to receive more love, affectionate pats, hugs, and snuggles is to be proactive and consistently demonstrate your genuine love and warmth to your significant other. Like your relentlessly adoring and affectionate pup, you may have to be doggedly determined and even resort to begging at times. Just keep at it and in no time you will find that it pays off as reliably well for you as it does for your dog.

Touch also plays a vital role in keeping two people together. Oxytocin is a hormone that has been dubbed the "cuddle-chemical." Childbirth and nursing powerfully stimulate the release of oxytocin, but so can hugging and hand-holding. Even watching romantic movies can cause the oxytocin levels of both men and women to rise. We suspect that someday we may be able to predict the popularity of a "chick-flick" by the average rise in oxytocin after viewing the movie.

Look Great Naked is the title of a best-selling diet and exercise book by Brad Schoenfeld. Sex, like the swimsuit season, can be a great motivator to stay fit, healthy, and attractive. And regular sex, like exercise, provides a boost to your self-esteem and mood. Sex does qualify as exercise. However, to burn off the 250 calories contained in a small candy bar, you would have to have vigorous sex for about two hours, which seems a little overly optimistic even in the age of Viagra. Still, any exercise is better than none, and sexual relations are generally a fun way to get your heart rate up. An active sex life not only helps married couples stay together and in love but is also one of the best predictors of someone who will stay young despite the passing years. Studies consistently show that one of the characteristics often found in men and women who are aging well is an interest in sex and regular sexual activity. Sex hormones, such as testosterone in males and estrogens in females and DHEA in both genders, are important for maintaining a youthful appearance and energy level, and regular sex is a surprisingly effective means to keep your sex hormones in the youthful range. And just thinking about sex has been shown to increase testosterone levels and the growth rate of beards (thankfully, only in men). Oxytocin and DHEA are both released during orgasm and have been shown to speed the healing process in animals. A study involving 100 young adults found those who had sex once or twice weekly had higher levels of immunoglobulins (antibodies) than those who had less frequent sexual activity. Both DHEA and testosterone levels, when maintained up in the normal range, also seem to protect against heart attack.

Michael Roizen, MD, a leader in the field of staying young, highlights the importance of an active sex life in his excellent book *The Real Age Makeover,* published in 2004. Dr. Roizen writes, "Practice a lot of safe sex. The more orgasms you have a year, the younger you are. The average number of orgasms for American men is fifty-eight per year. Increasing the number through mutually monogamous or safe sex to 158 makes your Real Age at least eight years younger than your calendar age."

According to a widely quoted 1997 study of five Welsh villages, men who had the most orgasms (twice a week or more) had a 50 percent lower mortality than those who had the least. Furthermore, a dose response was apparent: the more orgasms, the lower the risk of dying. You might speculate that this finding was just a reflection that the men having the most sex were young and healthy, which is the real reason why they had a lower risk of death. However, this protective effect of frequent sex was apparent even after statistically controlling for age, social class, smoking, blood pressure, and health status at baseline. In other words, no matter how old you are or what your other risk factors are, an active sex life (as long as it is safe sex) seems to be good for your health.

A more recent study published in April 2004 in the *Journal of the American Medical Association* by Dr. Michael Leitzmann followed more than 29,000 middle-aged men. It showed that for every three ejaculations per month during their adult life span, the risk of prostate cancer was lowered by about 15 percent. For men who reported twenty-one or more ejaculations per month across a lifetime, the relative risk of prostate cancer was 33 percent lower than those who reported four to seven ejaculations per month. Frequent sexual activity has also been linked to a lower rate of breast cancer in women, and improved overall longevity in both genders.

Studies also show that a divorce carries as much cardiovascular risk as smoking a pack of cigarettes a day. If you want a real recipe for heart attack, get a divorce and take up smoking at the same time. Researchers report that it is not marriage per se that leads to happiness and improved health. The same benefits are noted in single people who report having one or more close confidants.

An Improved Sex Life: Yet Another Benefit of Exercise

Regular exercise has been shown to improve your sex life. Scientific studies consistently find that aerobic exercise of forty-five minutes or more daily will usually lead to increased sexual desire in both genders and improvement in erectile dysfunction (ED) for males. Studies show a direct correlation between a man's waist size and his risk of erectile dysfunction—the bigger the waist the higher the likelihood of problems with impotence.

Erectile dysfunction is usually caused by poor blood flow to the penis, and new research indicates that it may be an early sign of heart disease. In a study published in the December 11, 2004, issue of the *British Medical Journal*, men with erectile dysfunction were eight times more likely to have blockage in their coronary arteries than those without ED.

The same principle holds for women—those who exercise regularly tend to have better sexual function. One study found that physically fit women had almost a twofold increase in blood flow to the vagina and labia when watching an erotic video compared to inactive women.

In contrast, stress chemicals and hormones can cause or worsen ED in men and impair a woman's ability to achieve orgasm. So activities resulting in a more relaxed state of mind and body can also benefit your sexual health.

Hormone Supplements

Recently one of my retired male patients told me this joke: An old gent picks up a frog, and it talks to him, saying, "If you kiss me I will turn into a beautiful princess." The man looks at the frog momentarily before putting it in his pocket. The frog croaks, "Wouldn't you like to have a beautiful princess at your service?" The man answers, "Frankly, at my age, I'd rather have a talking frog."

Male menopause, more appropriately referred to as andropause, is the result of falling testosterone levels. It often begins between the ages of forty and fifty, when the testosterone levels in men gradually start to decline. By age eighty, about 45 percent of men have low blood levels of testosterone by younger men's standards. Andropause is hastened by smoking, drinking alcohol excessively, obesity, eating the standard unhealthy American diet, and leading a sedentary lifestyle. Loss of interest in sex is just one of the symptoms of andropause, along with lethargy, depression, decreased brain function, irritability, decreased muscle mass and strength, increased fat especially in and around the belly, and erectile dysfunction. Testosterone supplementation to bring the levels back into the normal range is a great way to improve a man's quality of life. This is relatively easy to achieve by applying a small amount of Androgel (a prescription med) to the skin daily or receiving a monthly testosterone injection from your doctor. The benefits of testosterone therapy as reported by early trials include increased energy, libido, sexual function, muscle mass, brain function, and sense of well-being among men. There are potential risks, however, like worsening prostate enlargement, which are associated with testosterone replacement therapy and should be discussed with your physician.

The issue of female hormone supplementation is a controversial and confusing topic today. Scientifically rigorous trials of estrogen replacement therapy in postmenopausal women have increased the risk of breast cancer and abnormal blood clotting (predisposing to blood clots in the veins of the legs, heart attacks, and even strokes), and this is cause for concern. Still, estrogen does have benefits for the skin, brain, mood, and blood vessels. Whether we should use hormone replacement therapy or not remains an open question, and much more research will be needed before we know the final answer. We suspect that the right dose of the right female hormones would help to maintain youthfulness in women who are past menopause. For now, it would seem that using 17-Beta Estradiol, the precise hormone made by ovaries, in small doses is the safest choice for women who choose to take hormone replacement therapy. This is a highly individual decision that should be made by the woman and her physician after weighing the specifics of the family history, symptoms, current health, etc.

17

YOUR FAITH
CAN HEAL YOU

There are only two ways to live your life. One is as though nothing is a miracle.
The other is as though everything is a miracle.

—ALBERT EINSTEIN

In our dazzling, high-tech world, we sometimes forget that the discipline of medicine and healing is not just a science; it is an art as well. We are coming to understand, control, and even conquer diseases as we have never before been able to do. However, there will always be problems we cannot count on science alone to resolve. These are the times when many look for spiritual help. Such was the case for us about one and a half years into our marriage. Life was good. Joan was six months pregnant with our first child. We were out on a leisurely, carefree evening stroll when we noticed an unusual lump in her neck. The following morning a chest X-ray showed a malignant tumor the size of an orange in her chest with metastases in the lymph nodes under her right collarbone. One day we were worried about what color we should paint the baby's room, and the next we were worried about the chances of survival for Joan and our unborn baby. Our backs were to the wall as we stared into a frightening and uncertain future.

After a few long days and sleepless nights, we received the dreaded diagnosis of metastatic cancer, though thankfully a highly treatable form—Hodgkin's lymphoma.

Joan endured these soul-testing times like a trooper with unwavering resolve. She did exactly what her doctors recommended without moping or whining. Her strength to overcome what was to be a long, difficult road was rooted in a powerful faith. She knew that God was watching over her and her baby and that somehow, someday, everything would be all right again.

We prayed with all our might. Our families, friends, coworkers, and church all supported us with their prayers, too. Today, after nineteen years, and four pregnancies with four healthy children, she is still healthy and happy. We believe this is possible thanks to modern medicine, an excellent diet and lifestyle, and her unshakable faith.

> Sleep in peace, God is awake.
> —VICTOR HUGO

Your Innate Healing Power

Like Joan, you possess the ability to martial incredible strength and healing power from within your own minds and souls. To be honest, this power accounts for the popularity and effectiveness of physicians, healers, and medicine men down through the ages. Only for the past few decades have we physicians used therapies that really are effective in curing disease. One hundred years ago, if you came to us with a heart attack, we might have bled you with leeches, and it might have worked! If you truly believe you are going to get better, your chances of improving get better. Try as we might to explain these phenomena scientifically, they still largely remain a mystery.

Unfortunately, a dark side of the mind-body connections also exists. Incessant worries about future events that you can neither predict nor control can emotionally paralyze you. Chronic negative emotions like depression, loneliness, fear, hostility, and pessimism can take a toll on your health and impair your immunity and healing. Fear and anger are typical responses to a serious illness like heart disease or cancer. Negative emotions crank up your stress hormones, including adrenaline and cortisol, which are preparing you for fight or flight. These hormones may help you survive a sudden encounter with a mountain lion, but they hinder your immune system and are counterproductive when the threat is a chronic disease.

Faith can vanquish fear and other toxic emotions and harness the positive healing energy engendered by an optimistic and peaceful state of mind. Along with a network of social support, whether it be in the form of family, friends, community, or pets, faith can help sustain you and make you more resilient to stress and illness. Prayer and religious belief can also speed the healing process of virtually any disease.

Studies show people who have a faith or follow a religion, regardless of their denomination, tend to be healthier than those who don't participate in organized religion. A National Institute of Health (NIH) panel of physicians evaluated the evidence linking religion to health. This report published in the January 2003 *American Psychologist* journal reported a 25 percent lower risk of death in those who attended religious services at least once per week. Interestingly, watching religious services on TV conferred no health benefit. People who pray seem to recover from illness faster than those who do not.

Jesse Ventura, the outspoken former Minnesota governor, was quoted as saying, "Organized religion is a sham and a crutch for the weak-minded people who need strength in numbers." There will be times in our lives when each one of us will be weak or ill, and at those times the strength we draw from our faith and the support we receive from our circle of family, friends, and community may make the difference between life and death. When you nurture your spirit, it can be a real source of strength.

Do You Have a Prayer?

Harvard researchers surveyed more than 2,000 adults who were struggling with chronic, difficult-to-treat health issues like depression or back pain. Many people reported that they found that turning it over to a higher power was more helpful than a visit with the doctor.

What helped most for . . .	Prayer	Doctor
Severe depression	68%	48%
Anxiety	70%	38%
Arthritis	60%	40%
Back pain	59%	30%
Cancer	81%	78%

A disciplined cycle of flexing and then resting your muscles will enable you to grow strong and fit. The same sort of training can be used to improve the mental, emotional, and spiritual aspects of your life. Do what life demands of you, but make it a priority to cultivate your spirituality as well. Find time to pray or meditate daily. A few moments of solitude can keep you centered and in touch with your inner voice. Prayer and contemplation can create a sanctuary away from the noise and distractions that will help you discover and follow the path that is right for you.

When you ask for help from God, you tune into a spiritual force that just might be capable of providing an infinite supply of strength and support. The next time you are feeling hopeless, overwhelmed, or discouraged, try saying, "I pray for strength and guidance, please help me through this." The simple act of praying can provide remarkable improvements in your attitude and your health. Faith can heal; most scientists have accepted this much. How it works is a much more contentious issue. The placebo effect that helps to cure those patients who have faith in their doctors and therapies might also account for the health benefits of a belief in God. But does praying to God also tap into spiritual powers that dwell outside the realm of science and our physical universe?

The MAHI Prayer Study

A few years ago, a landmark trial from the Mid America Heart Institute was published in the June 2000 *Archives of Internal Medicine*, and it made national headlines. The Prayer Study, conceived by friend and colleague William Harris, PhD, was a randomized, controlled trial to answer the question, "Does intercessory prayer (praying for someone else) really make a difference in making people well again?"

About 1,000 patients who were admitted to the Heart Institute's Coronary Care Unit over a one-year period were randomly assigned to either prayer or no prayer. Those in the prayer group were prayed for individually for about twenty-eight days by groups of five volunteers. A total of seventy-five people in fifteen groups from a variety of denominations did the praying during the study. The patients were not aware of the study, nor were their doctors or other caregivers. The study was conducted silently and diligently, with the help of the chaplain's office at Saint Luke's Hospital in Kansas City.

At the end of the trial, those who were randomly assigned to the prayer group did significantly better and experienced 11 percent fewer adverse events and a 10 percent shorter stay in the CCU than those in the control group.

This was a scientifically sound, rigorously conducted trial that produced statistically significant benefits in favor of the people who were prayed for. The benefits might have been the result of chance alone, and other similar studies on intercessory prayer have produced mixed results. It seems unlikely that science will even definitely settle the issue of whether God answers prayer, or even exists. Nonetheless, if you find yourself beset by worries or feeling beleaguered and hopeless, try praying. It surely won't hurt, and it very well might help. Faith may not move mountains, but it certainly can help to bolster your spirits and rally your defenses to defeat illness.

It is said that God helps those who help themselves. Perhaps the most powerful advantage that prayer confers is a sense of optimism and strength. Turning a problem over to a higher power somehow unburdens you, enabling you to effectively mobilize the forces lying within your soul. Good old-fashioned faith and state-of-the-art medicine and are not incompatible. In fact, these two different strategies are synergistic. When used in tandem they provide a formidable defense against threats to your health and well-being—yet another example of the antiaging power of taking the best from both worlds.

**The wise man in a storm prays to God,
not for safety from danger, but for deliverance from fear.**
—RALPH WALDO EMERSON

18

LONGEVITY WITH SPIRIT: THE ART OF AGING GRACEFULLY

I will never be an old man. To me, old age is always fifteen years older than I am.

—Francis Bacon

James loves to ask his patients who are over ninety, "To what do you attribute your longevity?" They almost always have interesting insights like hard work, leading a clean life, getting out for fresh air and exercise every day, or choosing the right parents. The life expectancy of Americans has approximately doubled over the last century. The average American today lives seventy-eight years; males typically make it to age seventy-four, and females to age eighty. Scientists estimate the maximum potential human life span at 120 years, and in fact the longest well-documented human life was 122 years.

Longevity has been assumed to be mostly a matter of being born with the right genes, but experts tell us that only about one-third of aging is attributable to genetics. You have much more control over the aging process than you probably have imagined. Of course, you will age more gracefully if you exercise daily, maintain a healthy weight, eat right, and don't smoke or abuse alcohol. But learning how to effectively cope with and avoid stress is also a major factor in living a long and vigorous life. Among the strongest predictors of who will live to advanced ages are traits like optimism, volunteerism, and an ability to work through problems and still maintain enthusiasm and love of life.

Recently we celebrated the 102nd birthday of James's grandmother Dorothy O'Keefe. He lived with her for four years while he went to medical school, and she has always been an inspiration to him. Born in 1903, she came of age during the Roaring Twenties; the birth of her first child coincided with the onset of the Great Depression. She is an irrepressibly optimistic woman who, even today, is more interested in what is happening now than ruminating about days gone by. She did volunteer work well into her eighties, always has a drink or two of whiskey during happy hour, and has a zest for life. Dorothy is typical of the kind of person scientists tell us is likely to live a long life.

A recent study showed that people who live a century or more have several traits in common:

- A positive, yet realistic attitude
- An adventurous love of life
- A strong will
- Spiritual beliefs
- An ability to renegotiate life when necessary
- An insistence on aggressive medical care when necessary
- A sense of humor

The real beauty of these findings is that many of the same things that make life pleasurable—an ability to laugh, having faith, a happy outlook, a love of adventure, curiosity, and loving relationships—are the very same factors that will keep you alive and well for 100 years. Other characteristics of centenarians like strong will, the flexibility to renegotiate life, and willingness to find expert medical help when needed are crucial to overcoming the mental and physical maladies that we all develop sooner or later. About 80 percent of chronic serious medical conditions like heart disease, cancer, arthritis, Alzheimer's, diabetes, and so on are preventable with the right diet, lifestyle, attitudes, and medical care. Today more than ever, staying healthy is not a matter of fate, genes, or luck, but rather a function of your lifestyle and diet and how well you monitor your health and respond to the problems that will inevitably appear.

How to Stay Young

1. *Quit beating yourself up about things you can't change—like your age.*

2. *Spend time with your upbeat friends. The mopers will only drain the enthusiasm from your life.*

3. *Keep exploring. Never lose your enthusiasm for new people, places, and ideas. Do not let your mind idle. An idle brain is the Devil's workshop. And the Devil goes by the name Alzheimer.*

4. *Laugh out loud and laugh hard. Laugh until your sides hurt and you're gasping for breath.*

5. *Seize every opportunity to control your own life. The feeling that your life is out of your control leads to stress and aging. Maintaining a sense of control can help you weather stress like water off a duck's back.*

6. *Crises happen. Grieve, accept, adjust, and move on. The only person who is with you your entire life is you. Be gentle and forgiving with yourself. Do your best, and let it go.*

7. *Your home is your safe and comfortable refuge. Surround yourself with the passions and loves of your life, whether it's family, pets, gardens, or friends—connectedness and social relationships will buffer you from stress and prevent premature aging.*

8. *Safeguard your health: If it's strong, protect it. If you have issues (as we all do sooner or later), address them. Almost anything is fixable if you seek help for the problem rather than ignoring it.*

9. *Try to do the things you fear most. When you confront your inner demons, they lose their power over you. Fate often saves the warrior whose courage endures. Courage is an acquired skill, like a foreign language or golf, that can be mastered only through regular practice.*

10. *Skip the guilt trips. Take a trip to the lake, to the coast, even overseas; but NOT back to where the guilt lives. Regrets will take you nowhere but down.*

11. *Every chance you get, remind the people you love how special they are to you, and how much you love them. Cherish the moment; celebrate your chance to be alive now.*

Caroline, our five-year-old daughter, recently asked her great-grandmother Dorothy if she was old. Granny replied, "No honey, it's just that I've been young for a very long time." Perhaps the key to successful aging is not worrying about how long you live, but instead focusing on staying young and enjoying life in the meanwhile.

Never underestimate your power to change your life. Age per se does not undermine the ability to learn and grow and rejuvenate. Attitude, knowledge, and willpower are all you need to revolutionize your life. The human body is incredibly resilient. Even after years of abuse with a terrible diet, too much stress, not enough sleep, cigarettes, and too much alcohol and minimal exercise, many people still manage to live five or six decades. The body never functions optimally under these circumstances, but it sometimes manages to adapt to this unhealthy lifestyle and at least survive. One of the miracles of the human body, however, is its ability to heal itself when treated properly. The DNA in each of your cells remains largely unaltered, and the body can and will rejuvenate itself remarkably well if you begin to work with it rather than against it.

A ninety-one-year-old gentleman by the name of Sam Gadless is an inspirational example of the healing power of the body even after a lifetime of abuse. When Sam was in his seventies, his health was failing, and his doctor told him he did not have long to live. Now, twenty years later at age ninety-one, he competed in his seventh New York City marathon. He emigrated from Poland to America as a young man to escape the Holocaust and was a heavy smoker until he developed a life-threatening stomach ulcer that required surgery at age forty-five. By the time he was seventy, he had arthritis so severe he could not lift either arm above his head. His cholesterol and blood pressure were abnormally elevated, and he was a borderline diabetic. His doctor told him that his prognosis was very poor. "I was very unhealthy all of my life, and I don't have good genes. My father died when he was forty-two." How is it that Sam is still alive and running marathons twenty years later?

When Sam saw his life deteriorating into disability and suffering, he decided to do something about it. He became determined to take control of his health and his life. He began reading everything he could about preventing disease and living a healthy lifestyle. He also began to cook his own meals, avoiding high-fat meats, sugar, and white flour and instead opting for fruits, vegetables, grains, and modest amounts of red wine. He also enjoys salmon, sardines, and white tuna.

"I don't eat the bad stuff like milk shakes or the matzo ball soup my wife used to cook with butter or chicken fat." Instead, he is eating a sixteen-bean soup and "garlic by the pound." He trains by doing aerobics, stretching, and swimming, as well as light weight lifting, and he walks up to forty miles per week. He is not setting any records for the fastest time in the New York City marathon, but he is the oldest competitor. He has an irrepressible spirit and even had his left ear pierced for his ninetieth birthday. Sam says, "Age is just numbers. When I was younger, I was sick as could be. I am living my youth now."

It was not too late for Sam, and it is not too late for you. Your body will respond to an optimal lifestyle and mental attitude by healing illnesses and building strong new tissues. Dramatic healing like Sam experienced is possible but does not happen by coincidence. In order to allow your body to recover its vigor and vitality, you need to get smart about your diet and exercise program. Although he figured it out on his own, Sam has been following almost to the letter the Forever Young program. Many people have mixed emotions about living to an advanced age because they see images of old people who are disabled in nursing homes. But, if you could be enjoying life, attending parties, and competing in races, you probably would, like Sam and Granny, be happy to be alive at 100.

Dr. Leonard Poon from the University of Georgia has studied American centenarians since 1988. He refers to this select group as "expert survivors" and finds that they frequently share four coping mechanisms: They are practical, have a strong but flexible character, are relaxed in their approach to life, and tend to be independent thinkers who do not take information on a superficial level.

To stay healthy in our modern ultraconvenient world, you will also need to be a disciplined and motivated self-starter. A study from the University of California at Riverside found that conscientiousness was a personality trait shared by many people who live long and healthy lives. Whether you want to call it self-discipline, dependability, or the will to achieve, thinking about potential consequences before you act is critical for staying healthy and vigorous in the long term.

It's not that I'm afraid to die; I just don't want to be there when it happens.
—WOODY ALLEN

Longevity by the Numbers

Optimists on average live seven and a half years longer than pessimists.

Nonsmokers typically live ten years longer than smokers.

The people who typically sleep about seven to eight hours live longer than those who sleep less than five, or more than nine hours nightly.

Moderately tall people, men six feet to six three, and women five seven to five nine, live on average three years longer than shorter people.

Obesity will deduct seven years from the average woman's life expectancy and six years from a man's longevity.

Japanese live the longest, eighty-one years on average; Zambians live the shortest, at thirty-three years. Immigrants to the United States outlive native-born citizens by three years.

Oscar winners outlive the other nominees who did not win by four years. CEOs outlive corporate vice presidents.

For every one hour of exercise you do, you will live about two hours longer. For every sixty calories you eat above what you burn, you will shorten your life by one hour.

People who regularly attend worship services live seven years longer than those who do not.

Americans who receive higher education live on average six years longer than high-school dropouts.

Married people tend to outlive single folks by about three years, although men seem to benefit (or lose) more than women.

The average life expectancy for white Americans is eighty years, compared to seventy-five for African Americans. Much of that difference might be erased by good blood pressure control.

Remaining physically fit will add approximately seven years to your life.

For every ten points your systolic (top number) blood pressure is above 115, your chances of dying early increase by 30 percent. For every ten points of systolic blood pressure is lowered down toward 115, your chances of dying prematurely are decreased by 30 percent.

A sixty-five-year-old American woman can expect to live an additional twenty years; a sixty-five-year-old male can expect seventeen additional years.

Your odds of living to 116 years of age are 1 in 2 billion.

The simple recipe for a long and vigorous life is to concentrate on taking care of yourself so as to feel and look your best today. Laugh, play, be curious, stay physically active, eat whole fresh foods, drink water, sleep soundly, breathe deeply, love life, and invest yourself in the world around you. Life is for the living, and you are blessed with the gift of life today. In the final analysis, the mortality rate is 100 percent for everyone. So enjoy the moment; celebrate the opportunity to be a part of this wondrous world.

RESOURCES ON THE WEB

An ever-expanding array of Web sites is available on the Internet that can help you get information about your health. Here are just a few resources that will help.

WebMD.com
About.com Health
theheart.org
mayoclinic.com
obesity.org
health.nih.gov
deniseaustin.com
DrWeil.com
lef.org

INDEX